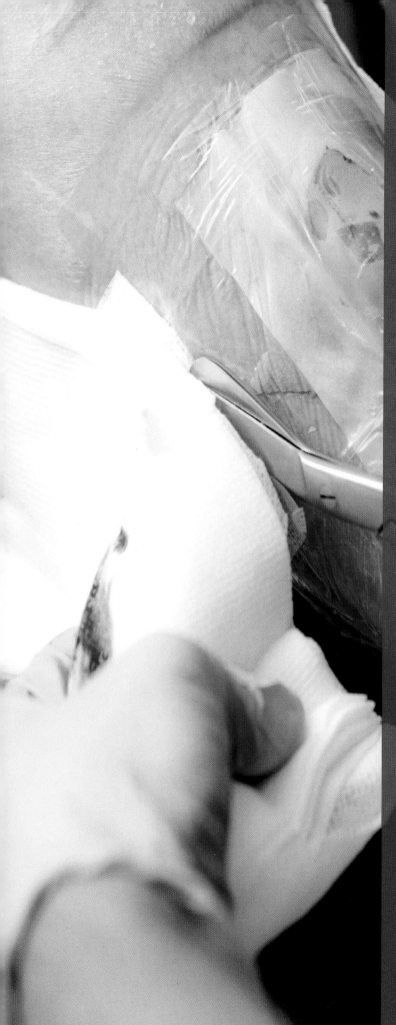

Wound Care
at a Glance

Ian Peate

EN(G) RGN DipN (Lond) RNT BEd (Hons) MA (Lond) LLM

Professor of Nursing, Head of the School of Health Studies, Gibraltar and Editor in Chief, British Journal of Nursing

Wyn Glencross

EN(G) RGN MA (LLM)

V300 Non-medical Prescribing; Member of the Expert Witness Institute

Independent Tissue Viability Nurse Consultant and Expert Witness

Series Editor: Ian Peate

WILEY Blackwell

This edition first published 2015 © John Wiley & Sons Ltd.

Registered Office
John Wiley & Sons Ltd, The Atrium, Southern Gate, Chichester, West Sussex, PO19 8SQ, UK

Editorial Offices
350 Main Street, Malden, MA 02148-5020, USA
9600 Garsington Road, Oxford, OX4 2DQ, UK
The Atrium, Southern Gate, Chichester, West Sussex, PO19 8SQ, UK

For details of our global editorial offices, for customer services, and for information about how to apply for permission to reuse the copyright material in this book please see our website at www.wiley.com/wiley-blackwell.

Library of Congress Cataloging-in-Publication Data
Peate, Ian, author.
  Wound care at a glance / Ian Peate, Wyn Glencross.
     p. ; cm. – (At a glance series)
  Includes bibliographical references and index.
  ISBN 978-1-118-68467-2 (pbk.)
  I. Glencross, Wyn, author. II. Title. III. Series: At a glance series (Oxford, England)
  [DNLM: 1. Wound Healing–Handbooks. 2. Wounds and Injuries–nursing–Handbooks. WO 39]
  RD93
  617.1 – dc23
                              2014032710

A catalogue record for this book is available from the British Library.

Cover image: iStock / © KarenMower

Set in 9/11pt Minion by Laserwords Private Limited, Chennai, India
Printed and bound in Singapore by Markono Print Media Pte Ltd

3   2017

Wound Care
at a Glance

This title is also available as an e-book.
For more details, please see
www.wiley.com/buy/9781118684672
or scan this QR code:

Contents

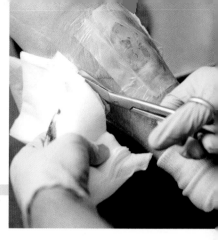

Part 5 **Dressing selection 53**

Part 6 **Complexities of wound care 69**

Preface

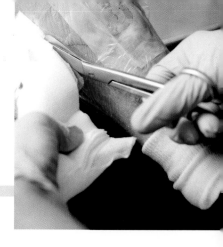

Wound care management continues to develop, requiring the nurse to respond to the needs of people as well as responding to the many technological advances being made. This is a dynamic and ever changing field. The nurse needs to keep up to date with regards to wound care in order to ensure that care provision is safe and effective.

Sustaining a wound that requires the needs of a nurse or healthcare provider who is conversant with wound care can occur to people across their lifespan, from all socioeconomic backgrounds and is prevalent in all care specialities and communities. The breakdown of skin can have a considerable impact on an individual, the individual's family and society, physically, psychologically and economically. There is a high probability that the person's health and wellbeing will be affected should they experience an adverse problem with skin integrity.

Successful advancement of the wound-healing discipline depends on effective integration of scientific discoveries and wound care practices. The science of wound healing is heavily interdisciplinary in nature.

Keeping abreast with the latest developments in the science of wound care can be a overwhelming task. *Wound Care at a Glance* is a compilation of key issues regarding wound care that nurses will find useful in ensuring that the patient is at the centre of all they do.

This book, in line with the *At A Glance* series, provides an accessible yet comprehensive discussion of key issues for nurses and other health care professionals helping them build on their knowledge and understanding of wound care with the overall aim of encouraging the reader to offer safe, effective and patient-centred care.

The book has been divided into six parts beginning with the history of wound care, the anatomy and physiology, the normal and abnormal healing process. The section in the book on wound management in practice describes the assessment of skin and the classification of wounds; in this section chapters are dedicated to the ethico-legal aspects of wound care along with treatment options and pain management. Dressing selection is a complex process and requires the nurse to bring together knowledge and understanding of the person and the myriad dressings available. Chapters that consider dressing selection and the factors that need to be taken into account when choosing an appropriate wound care product are discussed; there is an emphasis throughout on ensuring that individual needs are met. The final section of the text considers wound care complexities and discusses a range of situations that the nurse may face.

We have enjoyed writing this text and hope that by reading it you will be able enhance your current knowledge and understanding of wound care.

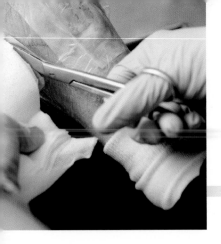

Acknowledgements

Ian would like to thank his partner Jussi Lahtinen for his support and Mrs Frances Cohen for her ongoing assistance . Wyn would like to thank Maureen Benbow, Senior Tissue Viability Lecturer at Chester University, for supplying a photograph used in the book. The authors would also like to thank Phil Vong for allowing use of his graphics and Katrina Rimmer at John Wiley and Sons for her assistance and guidance.

The following publications are acknowledged for granting permission for use of material:

Davey P (2014). *Medicine at a Glance*, 4e. John Wiley & Sons, Ltd, Oxford.

Grey JE, Harding KG, Enoch S (2006). ABC of wound healing: Pressure ulcers. *BMJ*;332:472–475. Figure 5, p. 473.

Keast DH, Bowering CK, Evans AW, Mackean GL, Burrows C, and D'Souza L (2004). MEASURE: A proposed assessment framework for developing best practice recommendations for wound. *Wound Rep Reg*;12:S1–S17.

Lawenda BD, Mondry TE and Johnstone, PAS (2009). Lymphedema: A primer on the identification and management of a chronic condition in oncologic treatment. *CA Cancer J Clin*; 59:8–24.

Nair M. and Peate I. (2013). *Fundamentals of Applied Pathophysiology*, 2e. John Wiley & Sons, Ltd, Oxford.

Onesti MG, Fino P, Fioramonti P, Amorosi V and Scuderi N (2013). Ten years of experience in chronic ulcers and malignant transformation. *Int Wound J*; doi:10.1111/iwj.12134.

The Malnutrition Advisory Group (2004). *Malnutrition Universal Screening Tool*. BAPEN, Redditch.

Thompson M and Van den Bruel A (2011). *Diagnostic Tests Toolkit*. John Wiley & Sons, Ltd, Oxford.

Timmons J (2006). Skin function and wound healing physiology. *Wound Essentials*: 1.

Ward JPT and Linden RWA (2013). *Physiology at a Glance*, 3e. John Wiley & Sons, Ltd, Oxford.

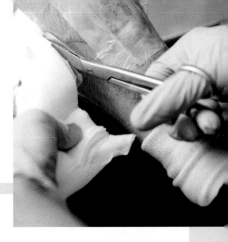

How to use your textbook

Features contained within your textbook

Each topic is presented in a double-page spread with clear, easy-to-follow diagrams supported by succinct explanatory text.

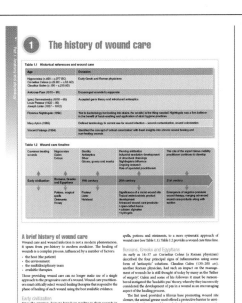

The website icon indicates that you can find accompanying resources on the book's companion website.

Your textbook is full of **photographs, illustrations and tables.**

Figure 21.1 Five stages associated with evidence-based practice

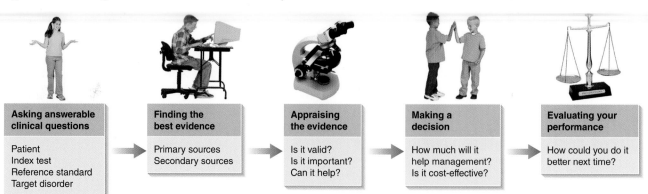

Asking answerable clinical questions	Finding the best evidence	Appraising the evidence	Making a decision	Evaluating your performance
Patient Index test Reference standard Target disorder	Primary sources Secondary sources	Is it valid? Is it important? Can it help?	How much will it help management? Is it cost-effective?	How could you do it better next time?

Source: Thompson and Van den Bruel 2011, figure on p. x of Introduction. Reproduced with permission of Wiley & Sons, Ltd.

Table 21.1 Hierarchy of evidence

Level	Description of evidence	Strength
I	Systematic review or meta-analysis of all relevant randomized controlled trials (RCTs), or evidence-based clinical practice guidelines based on systematic reviews of RCTs	Strongest
II	Evidence from at least one well-designed RCT	
III	Evidence from well-designed controlled trials without randomization	
IV	Evidence from well-designed case-control and cohort studies	
V	Systematic reviews of descriptive and qualitative studies	
VI	A single descriptive or qualitative study	
VII	The opinion of authorities and/or reports of expert committees	Weakest

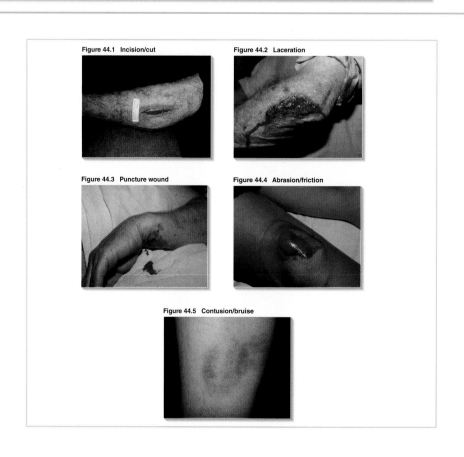

Figure 44.1 Incision/cut

Figure 44.2 Laceration

Figure 44.3 Puncture wound

Figure 44.4 Abrasion/friction

Figure 44.5 Contusion/bruise

About the companion website

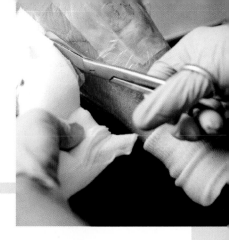

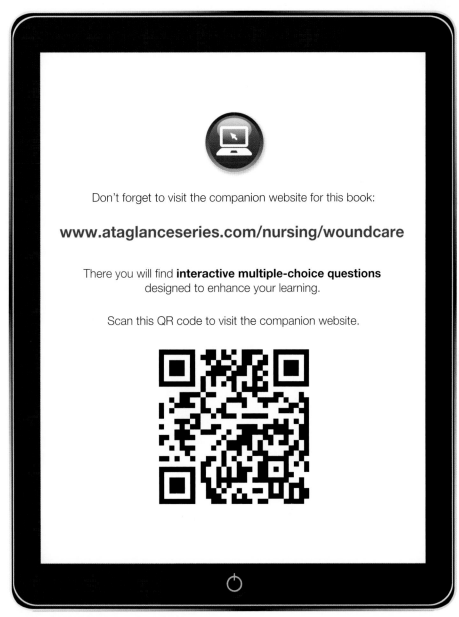

Don't forget to visit the companion website for this book:

www.ataglanceseries.com/nursing/woundcare

There you will find **interactive multiple-choice questions** designed to enhance your learning.

Scan this QR code to visit the companion website.

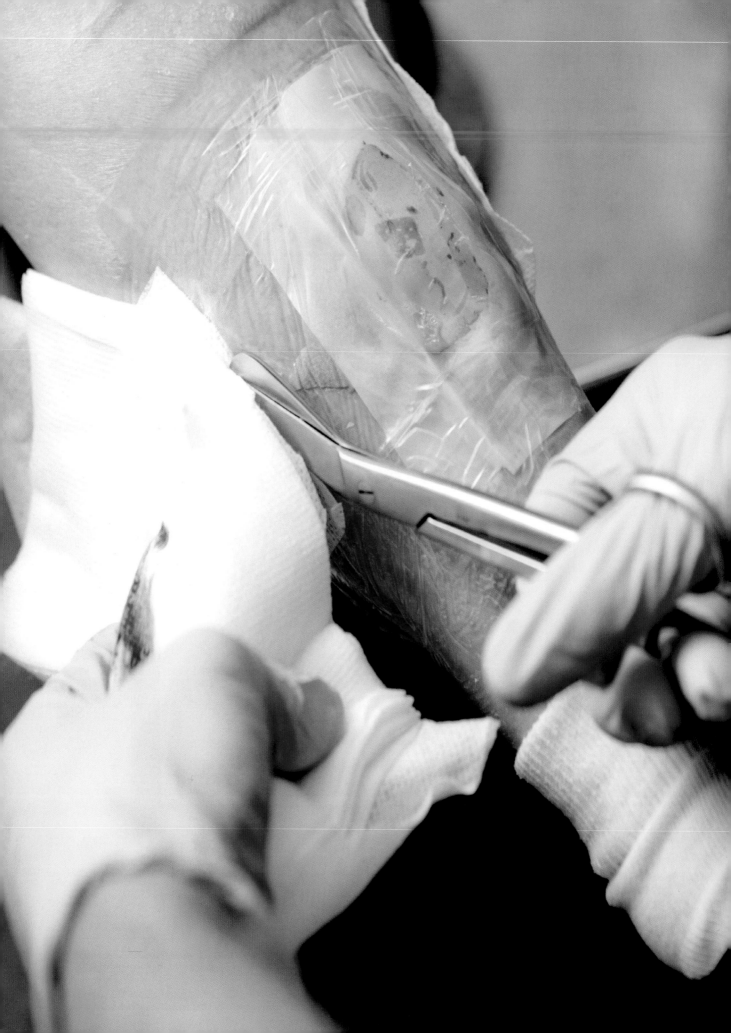

Anatomy and physiology

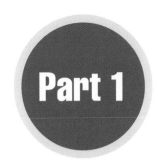

Part 1

Chapters

 Visit the companion website at www.ataglanceseries.com/nursing/woundcare to test yourself on these topics.

The history of wound care

Table 1.1 Historical references and wound care

Age	Occasion
Hippocrates (c.460 – c.377 BC) Cornelius Celsus (c.25 BC – c.50 AD) Claudius Galen (c.130 – c.210 AD)	Early Greek and Roman physicians
Ambrose Pare (1510 – 90)	Encouraged wounds to suppurate
Ignaz Semmelweiss (1818 – 65) Louis Pasteur (1822 – 95) Joseph Lister (1827 – 1912)	Accepted germ theory and introduced antiseptics
Florence Nightingale (1894)	'Not in bacteriology but looking into drains (for smells) is the thing needed'. Nightingale was a firm believer in the benefit of hand-washing and application of strict hygiene practices
Mary Ayton (1985)	Defined terminology in current use for wound infection – wound contamination, wound colonization
Vincent Falanga (1994)	Identified the concept of 'critical colonization' with fresh insights into chronic wound healing and non-healing wounds

Table 1.2 Wound care timeline

Cavemen treating wounds	Hippocrates Galen Celsus	Sterility Antiseptics Silver Gloves, gowns and masks	Fleming antibiotics Industrial revolution development of absorbent dressings Nightingale's influence Ongoing research Role of specialist practitioners	The role of the expert tissue viability practitioner continues to develop
Early civilization	**Romans, Greeks and Egyptians**	**19th century**	**20th century**	**21st century**
	Potions, magical spells Ointments Honey	Pasteur Lister Halstead	Significance of a moist wound site Topical antimicrobials product development Advanced wound care products: • open-celled foams • calcium alginates • hydrogels	Emergence of negative pressure wound therapy, merging advanced wound care products along with suction

Wound Care at a Glance, First Edition. Ian Peate and Wyn Glencross. © 2015 John Wiley & Sons, Ltd. Published 2015 by John Wiley & Sons, Ltd.
Companion website: www.ataglanceseries.com/nursing/woundcare

A brief history of wound care

Wound care and wound infection is not a modern phenomenon, it spans from pre-history to modern medicine. The healing of wounds is a complex process, influenced by a number of factors:

- the host (the patient)
- the environment
- the multidisciplinary team
- available therapies.

Those providing wound care can no longer make use of a single approach to the progressive care of a wound. Wound care practitioners must critically select wound-healing therapies that respond to the phase of healing of each wound using the best available evidence.

Early civilization

Since the caveman, humans have been tending to their wounds in one form or another. Wound care continues to evolve from magical spells, potions and ointments, to a more systematic approach of wound care (see Table 1.1). Table 1.2 provides a wound care time line.

Romans, Greeks and Egyptians

As early as 14–37 AD Cornelius Celsus (a Roman physician) described the four principal signs of inflammation using some form of 'antiseptic' solutions. Claudius Galen (130–200 AD), another Roman physician, had such an impact on the management of wounds he is still thought of today by many as the 'father of surgery'. Galen and some of his followers it must be remembered instigated the 'laudable pus' theory, whereby they incorrectly considered the development of pus in a wound as an encouraging aspect of the healing process.

The lint used provided a fibrous base promoting wound site closure, the animal grease used offered a protective barrier to environmental pathogens and honey helped as its actions were antimicrobial. Egyptians and the Greeks observed the significance of closing a wound. The Greeks were the first to make a difference between acute and chronic wounds, correspondingly calling them 'fresh' and 'non-healing'. Around 120–201 AD, a Greek surgeon who served Roman gladiators made a number of contributions to wound care, recognizing how important it was to maintain a wound site that was moist helping it to close successfully.

After the fall of the Roman Empire these many advances were lost. In the Middle Ages in Europe there was a regression of wound care returning to the use of potions and charms.

The use of honey as a wound care treatment has recently seen a revival. Ancient Egyptians used honey as a wound treatment as early as 3000 BC and it has been found in Egyptian tombs. Honey is said to have been an essential aspect of the 'Three Healing Gestures' used by the Egyptians.

19th century

Pasteur's theories associated with the impact of microbes on disease and Lister's use of phenol introduced the modern 'germ theory' when he demonstrated the beneficial effects of carbolic acid (phenol) in the dressings of infected wounds at the turn of the century. Halstead introduced the wearing of gloves, gowns and masks and silver was revived as an antiseptic used in dressings, enhancing the healing of wounds.

All of these events make the 19th century a significant and eventful era with regards to advances within the field of sterility and sterile surgical procedures. Skin cleaning, the use of antiseptics and debridement became common practices thereafter.

20th century

The 20th century brought with it key advances when there was a resurgence and rediscovery of the significance of a moist wound site with the invention and development of polymer synthetics used for wound dressings.

Fleming's discovery and the subsequent development of antibiotics provided us with potent antimicrobial therapies with high specificity, transforming clinical therapy marking the decline of a number of former remedies. Yet, the emergence of antibiotic resistant strains of pathogens, alongside the delayed discovery of newer antibiotics led to a need for the discovery and development of alternative treatments.

Topical antimicrobials in current wound care practice included: iodine and silver containing products. In the past acetic acid, chlorhexidine, hydrogen peroxide, sodium hypochlorite, potassium permanganate and proflavine have been used. Some are making a come back, other options are being investigated and considered.

In the UK during the 1800s, natural products were being refined leading to the development of absorbent natural products for dressings including spun and woven cotton. Plastics were being added to cotton in the 1950s creating composite dressings such as plasters. Throughout this timeframe, the key aim was to dry out the wound, focusing upon protection and absorption, reducing the trauma of dressing changes. There is much evidence to suggest that keeping wounds moist is more effective to letting them dry out.

Advanced wound care products were being designed in the 1970s taking advantage of this concept; nurses were using these products to successfully treat chronic wounds. Much research was undertaken in the late 1970s and 1980s.

Early 1980s the second advanced dressing, the hydrocolloid was developed. Hydrocolloid wafers were established as first-line treatment for pressure ulcers, leading to the development of more absorbent dressings, for example foams and alginates.

The late 1980s witnessed the introduction of other advanced wound care products:

- open-celled foams
- calcium alginates
- hydrogels

Nurses began to take the lead with wound care or tissue viability managing and organizing, outpatient wound clinics, influencing and enhancing patient care.

Product diversification and growth continued throughout the 1990s. Sustained-release antimicrobial dressings were beginning to emerge and growth factor impregnated hydrogel and living skin equivalents.

21st century

Throughout the 2000s, product modification continues and this will continue with the emergence of negative pressure wound therapy, merging advanced wound care products along with suction.

The future

The field of medicine is constantly evolving including the field of wound care. A number of new laboratory tools have provided us with the ability to gather an incredible amount of scientific data as to the biological events associated with healing. Much more needs to be accomplished, pieces of the jigsaw are still missing, fitting together in a way that is important for the patient. The future is unknown but, people requiring wound care will need still need treatment that is kind and compassionate.

2 Anatomy and physiology of the skin

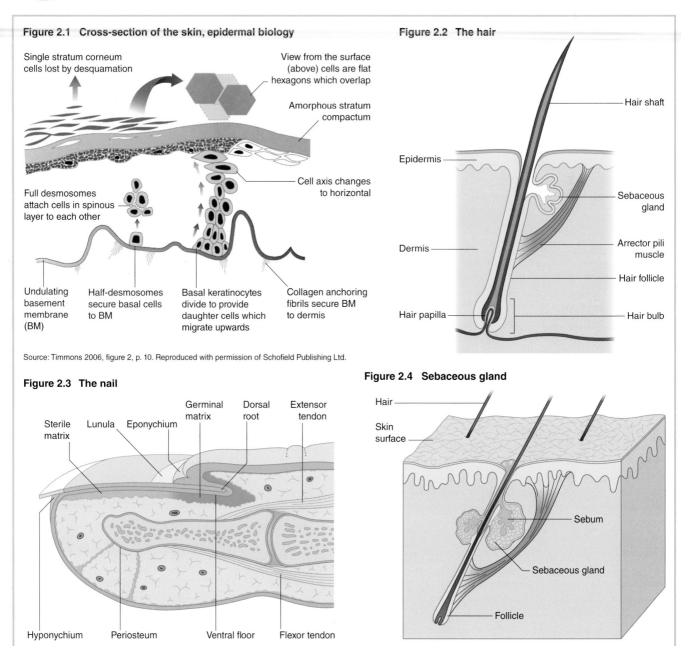

Figure 2.1 Cross-section of the skin, epidermal biology

Single stratum corneum cells lost by desquamation

View from the surface (above) cells are flat hexagons which overlap

Amorphous stratum compactum

Cell axis changes to horizontal

Full desmosomes attach cells in spinous layer to each other

Undulating basement membrane (BM)

Half-desmosomes secure basal cells to BM

Basal keratinocytes divide to provide daughter cells which migrate upwards

Collagen anchoring fibrils secure BM to dermis

Source: Timmons 2006, figure 2, p. 10. Reproduced with permission of Schofield Publishing Ltd.

Figure 2.2 The hair

Hair shaft

Epidermis

Sebaceous gland

Dermis

Arrector pili muscle

Hair follicle

Hair papilla

Hair bulb

Figure 2.3 The nail

Sterile matrix

Lunula

Eponychium

Germinal matrix

Dorsal root

Extensor tendon

Hyponychium

Periosteum

Ventral floor

Flexor tendon

Figure 2.4 Sebaceous gland

Hair

Skin surface

Sebum

Sebaceous gland

Follicle

Wound Care at a Glance, First Edition. Ian Peate and Wyn Glencross. © 2015 John Wiley & Sons, Ltd. Published 2015 by John Wiley & Sons, Ltd.
Companion website: www.ataglanceseries.com/nursing/woundcare

The skin is the largest organ of the body and consists of accessory organs: glands, hair and nails (the appendages). It is a multifunctional organ:

- protection against biological invasion, physical damage and ultraviolet radiation
- sensation provided by nerve endings
- provides thermoregulation provided through sweating and regulation of blood flow
- synthesis of vitamin D
- sweat excretes salts and small amounts of waste
- aesthetics and communication.

The skin has three layers: the epidermis (Figure 2.1), the demis and the hypodermis. Skin health has a great impact on the overall health of the individual and is of profound psychological importance.

Epidermis

This consists mainly of stratified epithelium, the outer layer, continually shedding dead cells, slightly acidic pH 4.5–6. The basal layer is constantly forming new cells gradually moving towards the surface and flattening during this process prior to being shed from the surface of the skin; can take between 28 and 35 days. Depending on their location, these cells are normally four or five layers thick, the most layers present on the palms and the soles.

Layers of the epidermis
The epidermis is divided into five layers: stratum corneum, stratum lucidum, stratum granulosum, stratum spinosum, stratum basale.

Stratum corneum Tough, waterproof uppermost layer, consisting of fibrous dead cells, assists with the maintenance of pH and temperature and plays a protective role. The continual replacement of the millions of worn out cells contribute to skin's ability to repair itself.

Stratum lucidum Not always present in some areas of the body, where skin is thinner. Provides extra protection in those areas exposed to wear and tear.

Stratum granulosum In this layer keratinocytes lose their nuclei and start to flatten and die, keratinization takes place in this layer. The stratum granulosum helps reduce loss of water from the epidermis.

Stratum spinosum Contains living cells with spiny processes called desmosomes. The stratum spinosum is 8–10 cells thick.

Stratum basale Also known as the basement membrane, this is the lowest layer. It is one cell thick and forms a definitive border between the dermis and the epidermis. Cells at this level are continually dividing and developing providing ongoing rejuvenation of the skin.

Melanocytes are produced here.

Dermis

The key purpose is to support and provide nutrition to the epidermis.

The key component of the dermis is proteinous connective tissue made up of arc shaped elastic fibres, undulated and practically inelastic, collagen fibres (elastin). Other constituents include: fibroblasts, mast cells, other tissues cells, multiple blood and lymph vessels, nerve endings, hot and cold receptors, tactile sensory organs.

It contains blood capillaries, sensory nerve endings, lymphatic vessels, sweat glands, sebaceous glands and hair follicles.

The flexible irregular connective tissue made from woven collagen and elastin fibres abound with blood vessels, nerve fibres and lymphatic vessels. Ridges formed from these bundles of collagen run downward, forward and horizontally around the body and are named cleavage lines and are genetically determined and are unique for each person.

Hypodermis
The superficial facia provides anchorage to the skin while allowing some capacity for it to move. Offers support to the dermis and is made up primarily of: adipose tissue, connective tissue, blood vessels. The fat stored within the hypodermis offers protection to the internal structures and insulates against cold.

Appendages

Hair
Made up of keratin, at the lower end is a bulb or root that is enclosed in a follicle that produces the hair. The root is indented by a hair papilla, connective tissue and blood vessels. The hair follicle is an epithelium lined sheath, the arrector pilli (smooth muscle) extends through the dermis and attaches to the base of the follicle, hair stands on end when muscle contracts (Figure 2.2).

On the palms of the hands, soles of the feet, nails, parts of the external genitals, lips and nipples do not have hair. Key function is protection. Protection of the skin by hair is constrained; however its role is to protect the scalp specifically from the ultraviolet rays, heat loss and injury. The eyebrows and the eyelashes provide protection from foreign bodies entering the eye.

Nails
The nails are specialized types of keratin and are situated over the distal surface of fingers and toes. The nail plate is surrounded on three ends by cuticles. (see Figure 2.3).

The function of nails is to assist with the development of fine motor skills such as grasping, scratching and manipulation. It provides protection against trauma to the fingers and toes.

Sebaceous glands
These are located on all parts of the skin except palms; they are more prominent on the scalp, face, upper torso and genitalia, producing sebum, made up of keratin, fat and cellulose debris. Sebum forms a moist, oily acidic film that has antibacterial and antifungal properties (Figure 2.4).

Blood vessels
Blood vessels include arterioles, capillary networks and venules. Blood vessels in the skin are responsible for the transportation and distribution oxygen, nutrients and hormones as well as the removal of waste products.

Nerve fibres
Within the dermis there are both sensory and motor nerves. The sensory nerve endings are sensitive to touch, or initiate signals producing sensations of warmth, coolness, pain, pressure, vibration, tickling and also itching.

Lymphatic vessels
The lymphatic system matches the blood vessels supply and function.

Figure 3.1   Changing Faces campaign poster

The skin – psychological and social

The physical presence of the skin as the largest organ of the body is significant in relation to a person from psychological and social perspectives. The skin has psychological and social components; it can lead to discrimination and has the ability to reveal how we are from a health and wellbeing perspective. The interplay between the skin and the mind and the individual has been the subject of study for many years. When practitioners understand this complex relationship they will then be able to provide assistance with regards to the various coping mechanisms that can be used by people to help them live with wounds – healed or healing. Self-harm and how this manifests and can be treated is addressed in Part 6.

Stress and anxiety

Psychological stress and physiological stress (for what ever reason) can change the wound healing process. Psychological stress can have a significant, clinical impact on wound repair.

Wound-healing processes can be directly impacted on by the physiological stress response whereas psychological stress can impact indirectly resulting in a modification of the repair process, this may occur by the promotion of health-damaging behaviours being adopted by the patient.

Wound healing is an important aspect concerned with the recovery from injury and surgical interventions. If healing is negatively impacted upon this can increase the risk of:

- developing wound infections
- developing other complications
- increasing the duration of hospital stay
- increasing patient discomfort
- delaying the patient's ability to perform the activities of living and returning to independence.

A significant number of people suffer some form of psychological distress after they have sustained a wound or there has been damage to skin integrity. The person may experience the impact of an altered body image and this can lead the person to feel devalued by society as well as those close to them.

A wound in the process of healing or having healed resulting in scar formation can lead to the person believing that they are a 'social leper', whereby they feel others do not want to mix or be associated with them. The person's quality of life can be adversely affected.

Anxiety

Anxiety can be associated with a number of things, for example:

- uncertainty
- admission to hospital
- fear of pain
- fear of death
- fear of the unknown

While some degree of anxiety may be beneficial, excessive and prolonged anxiety can lead to psychological and physiological dysfunction. The Hospital Anxiety and Depression Score can be used to help identify the levels of stress being experienced. The self-assessment results can help the practitioner and patient to formulate a plan that will assist in relieving the anxiety and stress being experienced.

Practitioners should consider assessing and reassessing the patient's psychological state as part of the overall plan of care. It is essential to make a baseline observation and compare consecutive observations with the baseline.

Emotional impact

As well as the physical discomfort often caused by wounds and the morbidity associated with them wounds also have an inherent emotional effect on the person, the people delivering care, family members, friends and onlookers. Wounds are often viewed negatively and patients may feel unattractive, vulnerable, contagious, imperfect and in some instances repulsive. Wounds can be seen as appalling, scary, time-consuming, costly, smelly, dirty, disfiguring, uncomfortable and unpleasant; they can cause people to feel humiliated, embarrassed, guilty and shamed. All of this can lead to extreme self-consciousness and social isolation

Management

A multidisciplinary approach is required. Competent psychological assessment demonstrates to the patient that they are valued and this can lead to positive health care outcomes. Management should include interventions that minimize patient distress, including the provision of social support and the development of coping skills. A psychosomatic approach should combine psychological therapy as well as physical therapy that consider the person holistically. The aim should be to eliminate pain if present, consider pharmacological interventions and the physical and psychological components, and must be tailored to each patient's needs. Failing to address issues such as pain can make depression worse and impact further on a person's self esteem.

Cognitive behavioural therapy

The psychological intervention that has the greatest evidence for success is cognitive behavioural therapy (CBT), which includes stress management, problem solving, meditation, relaxation and goal setting. In CBT, therapists help patients:

- with their communication skills
- provide a sense of control
- cope with the fear of pain and rejection.

This is done through learning positive coping strategies and will go some way to improving the person's mood.

CBT, a talking therapy, focuses on the here and now and aims to change thoughts and behaviours in order to improve mental health and wellbeing. The central principle of CBT is that it can change thought and behavioural patterns, having a significant impact on a person's emotions; this approach can help people identify and analyse any counter-productive thoughts and behaviours they may have. A skilled and trained therapist working with the person can help to ease feelings of anxiety or depression. CBT is recommended by the National Institute for Health and Care Excellence, which has provided guidelines for use that relate to disorders such as anxiety.

Referral

Appropriate referral may need to be made to other agencies such as a counsellor, psychotherapist or referral to external agencies within the third sector such as the charitable organization Changing Faces http://www.changingfaces.org.uk/ (Figure 3.1).

Body image

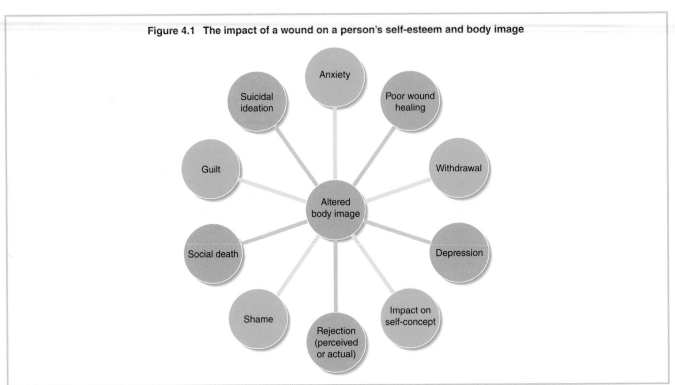

Figure 4.1 The impact of a wound on a person's self-esteem and body image

Body image

In contemporary Western societies appearance in general and specifically body image have become central and important concepts. The body beautiful and the strong emphasis on appearance are very much evident when media images are perused, shop windows are looked at, magazines flicked through and websites visited. The amount of money spent in the pursuit of beauty through dieting, aesthetic surgical procedures and everyday grooming practices reinforces the emphasis we place on appearance and appearance esteem.

The body image is associated with the mental representation or perception that we create of what we think it is we look like; it can or may not bear a close relation to how others really see us; this may be very different from a person's actual physical appearance. Body image is subjected to many different kinds of distortion that can come from internal factors such as our emotions, moods, our early experiences, the attitudes of our parents and more. However, it has a strong influence on behaviour. Infatuation with and distortions of body image are widespread among those people (as well as onlookers) who have a wound or have a scar that has formed as a result of a wound.

All those with wounds will experience some form of altered body image and this in turn can have an effect on the person's sense of self-esteem. The person's social and psychological wellbeing is in danger of being threatened and as such their quality of life can be impacted on in a negative and a detrimental way. Those wounds that result in disfigurement such as

- amputation
- mastectomy
- burns
- formation of ostomy

can profoundly alter the mental picture that the person has of him or her – their body image. This is confounded further as the person may be anxious about the unknown and their prognosis.

Disfiguring surgery such as mastectomy or amputation bring with it a dramatic change in body image; this coupled with the diagnosis of a life-threatening condition such as cancer can leave a person vulnerable. Those who have undergone disfiguring surgery with for example, the loss of a body part may be experiencing and going through the grieving process and having to deal with a number of mixed emotions such as:

- loss
- anxiety
- withdrawal of social relationships
- depression
- suicidal ideation.

Natural changes to body image such as the changes that are associated with puberty and ageing are generally expected changes, but the development from a wound may not be. Altered body image happens when unnatural or unexpected changes in a person's self-concept occur, for example a wound. Wounds can bring with them unexpected challenges and are themselves capable of changing the course of a person's life.

The circumstances, the visibility and the severity under which the injury occurred can have a significant effect on the person's acceptance of the wound associated with his or her altered body image (Figure 4.1). Some people have developed coping mechanisms that enable them to think that the wound does not belong to them (objectification).

Management

The response a person makes to the presence of a wound (patient, healthcare provider or stranger) is unpredictable. Those wounds that are present on the face, hands and neck are often the most difficult to conceal from the view of others as well as the person themselves

Assessing the impact of altered body image

Wound assessment should also take into account the assessment of the person's physical and psychological wellbeing as both may have negative impact upon the wound healing process (see Chapter 3).

Body image can be adversely affected or altered (temporarily or permanently) as a result of a change in the person's physical appearance such as trauma or the result of surgical intervention. Acute and chronic wounds have the potential to adversely impact on a person's body image and as such their self-esteem

There are a number of tools and scales that can be used to assess the impact of altered body image on a person. A five-point Likert scale has been developed – the Stigma Scale – that can be used to provide objectivity as to how the person views their body image. There are different types of stigma, for example:

- anticipated stigma (perceived stigma)
- internalized stigma (self-stigma)
- experienced stigma (discrimination).

When the results of the assessment are analysed, a care pathway can be formulated to help the person and their families cope with the problems and challenges they may have. The practitioner should aim to establish a person-centred approach that acknowledges the person as whole. Neglecting the psychological needs of the person may result in a threat to the person's quality of life and their sense of self. The emotional trauma experienced by people with wounds that result in an altered body image due to disfiguration can take many years of adjustment (and in some cases the person may never adjust to the degree of mutilation experienced).

Each change of dressing brings attention to the injured body part; brings with it pain and a reminder of the injury and how this occurred as well as possible fears about the future. The way a healthcare provider responds to a wound, for example, through acceptance, compassion, disappointment, repulsion, fear or avoidance can have a detrimental impact on the person's emotional state and their self esteem.

Referral

It may be necessary to make appropriate referrals to other agencies such as a counsellor or psychotherapist, or there may be a need to refer to external agencies where services such as skin camouflage can be offered to people who feel they need help to grow in confidence and independence.

The skin and ageing

Table 5.1 Wound healing and ageing skin

Effect of ageing on skin	Effect of ageing on healing
Keratinocyte maturation is decreased	Reduction in the ability of the skin to repair Wound contraction decreases
Reduction in the production of melanocytes	When exposed to the sun, reaction of the skin decreases
Merkel cell production is reduced	Sensation is reduced
Dermal/epidermal junction flattens	Likelihood of skin rupture increases resulting in skin tear Delivery of nutrients to the epidermis impaired Microcirculation diminished Possibility of an increase of shearing and blistering
Reduction in the number of Langerhans cells	Immune response inhibited or reduced
Diminished sebaceous and sweat gland activity and therefore reduction in the production of sebum	Dehydration of the skin Ability to maintain normal acidity compromised pH of the skin increases Uncharacteristic fissure formation, scaling, cracking and pruritis
The normal barriers of protection lose their effectiveness	Increased vulnerability to harmful irritants Increased vulnerability to developing contact dermatitis Transdermal permeability of water increases
Diminished sensory perception	Difficulty in being able to discern sensations increases
Decreased vascularity	Ability to thermoregulate effectively impaired Decrease in angiogenesis (capillary growth) Decreased ability to form granulation tissue Impairment in the supply of nutrients to the skin
Dermal atrophy	The skin's protective padding decreases A potential danger of damage and risk to underlying structures

Wound Care at a Glance, First Edition. Ian Peate and Wyn Glencross. © 2015 John Wiley & Sons, Ltd. Published 2015 by John Wiley & Sons, Ltd.
Companion website: www.ataglanceseries.com/nursing/woundcare

Ageing population

In the UK and other Western countries, there is an ageing population. The number of people over the age of 65 years is set to rise and continue to rise. Older skin brings with it many challenges related to intrinsic and extinct factors.

Skin changes are among the most visible signs of ageing. Evidence of increasing age includes wrinkles and sagging skin. Another obvious sign of ageing is the whitening or greying of the hair

At the cellular level

As we age, skin structure and its normal functions go through gradual change. As a result of these structural and functional changes, the ability of tissue to repair becomes impaired and processes alter. The ability of a wound to contract and for re-epithelialization to occur slows, the accumulation of connective tissue diminishes and ultimately wound tensile strength decreases. At each layer of the skin there are specific characteristic changes that occur as we age.

From a histological perspective (at cellular level) the epidermis is thinned along with a loss of the rete ridge and reduction in the amount of Langerhans cells and melanocytes; the remaining melanocytes increase in size. Ageing skin thus appears thinner, paler, and clear (translucent). Large pigmented spots (called age spots, liver spots, or lentigos) may appear in sun-exposed areas.

The epidermal cells reduce in size and the dermis becomes thinner, predominantly due to a loss of proteoglycans. From a functional perspective elasticity and tensile strength are reduced. Risk of damage from injury, irritants and infection is increased, and wound healing occurs at a slower rate. See Table 5.1 for a summary of the changes associated with the ageing skin.

The epidermis

The epidermis is in a constant state of change, with the production of new cells approximately every 28 days. The keratinocytes that are formed in the basement membrane go through chemical and morphological changes as they move through the epidermis, where they eventually shed to make way for a new layer of matured keratinocytes. The number of keratinocytes available to resurface and replace those lost cells decreases as we age. In the older person, the normal maturation rate of the epidermal macrophages – Langerhans cells – is decreased. As well as this, there is also a decrease in the number of cells that are required to fight off infections.

This decrease in the number of cells responsible and acting as first responders in relation to infection causes a diminished immune system response. As we age, the normal number of melanocytes that are present in the epidermis decreases; in addition, melanin production within the hair bulb is also changed.

The skin appendages are also affected by age. The nails also change with ageing. They grow slower and may become dull and brittle. They may become yellowed and opaque. Nails, particularly toenails, may become hard and thick. Ingrown toenails are more common. The tips of the fingernails may also fragment.

Hair loss does not decrease but the hair follicles become less dense and less active; hair colour changes as the follicle produces less melanin, hair loss occurs and the rate of hair growth changes. Many hair follicles stop producing hair altogether; hairs that remain may become coarser. There is dermal papillae flattening with the loss of the rete ridge, and this results in greater slippage between the epidermis and dermis (skin tears occur more easily). Sweat glands and sebaceous glands are less dense and as such less productive; the result is seen as a decrease in the hydration of the skin.

Dermis

Assessment of the older person's skin will reveal that it is thin, fragile and inelastic. The rates at which fibroblasts reproduce decreases and this reduced production leads to a scant and poorer quality of collagen production. With the loss of blood vessels this will mean that there will be a marked reduction in the rate of neoangiogenesis (new blood vessel growth). These two features together mean that there will be slower rates of granulation tissue growth and also a poorer quality granulation tissue. The blood vessels of the dermis become more fragile. This leads to bruising, bleeding under the skin (known as senile purpura), cherry angiomas and similar conditions. Raised collections of blood (haematomas) may form after even a minor injury has occurred.

Decreased elastin production results in decreased resilience of the skin as well as decreased resistance to external friction and shear forces. The ageing lymphatic system is less able to manage and maintain normal interstitial fluid levels.

Subcutaneous tissue

Consequences of a decrease in the amount of subcutaneous tissue are atrophy and fragile skin in the ageing person. Fragmenting of elastin results in the development of fibre networks forming fine wrinkles. Sensory perception is altered, resulting in a decreased ability to discriminate between heat, pain, vibration and itching, putting the older person at an increase risk of injury.

The subcutaneous fat layer thins, reducing normal insulation and padding. This increases the risk of skin injury and reduces the person's ability to maintain body temperature. As a result of the reduction in natural insulation, there is increased risk of hypothermia in cold weather.

The fat layer absorbs some medications and loss of the subcutaneous fat layer changes the way that these medications will work. The use of patch medication may need to be reconsidered.

Skin changes and loss of subcutaneous fat combined with a tendency to be less active as well as some nutritional deficiencies and other illnesses contribute to pressure ulcers. Ageing skin repairs itself more slowly than younger skin does. Wound healing can be up to four times slower. This contributes to pressure ulcers and infection. Diabetes, blood vessel changes, lowered immunity, and similar factors also affect healing.

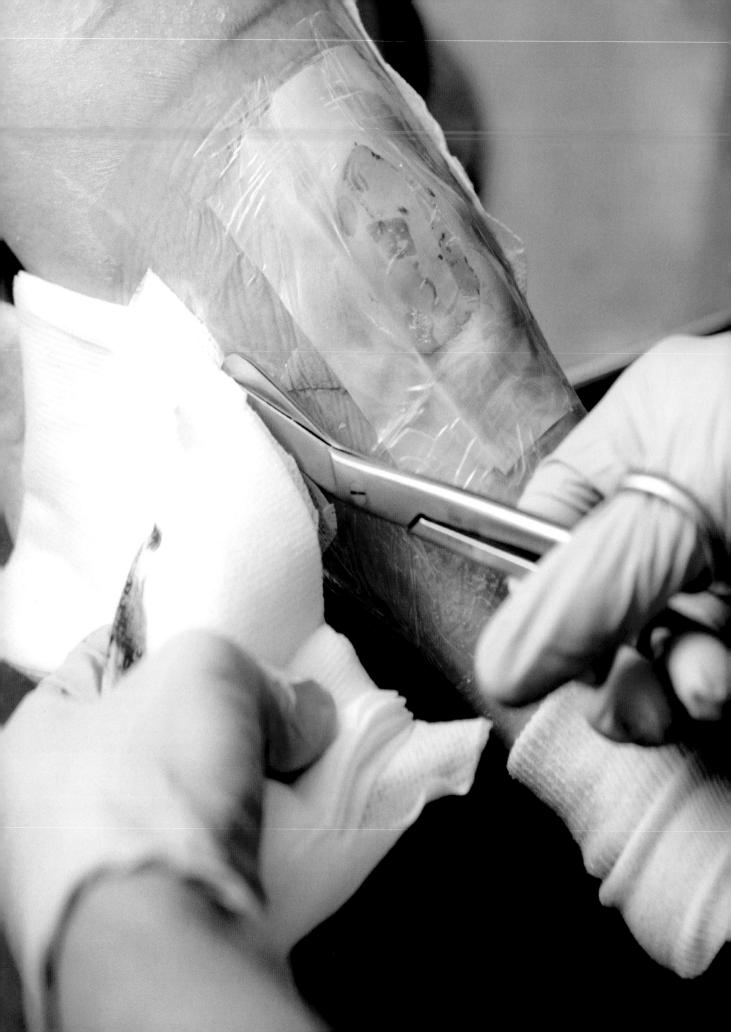

The normal healing process: acute wounds

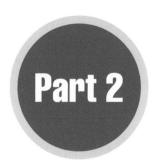

Part 2

Chapters

 Visit the companion website at www.ataglanceseries.com/nursing/woundcare to test yourself on these topics.

Haemostasis

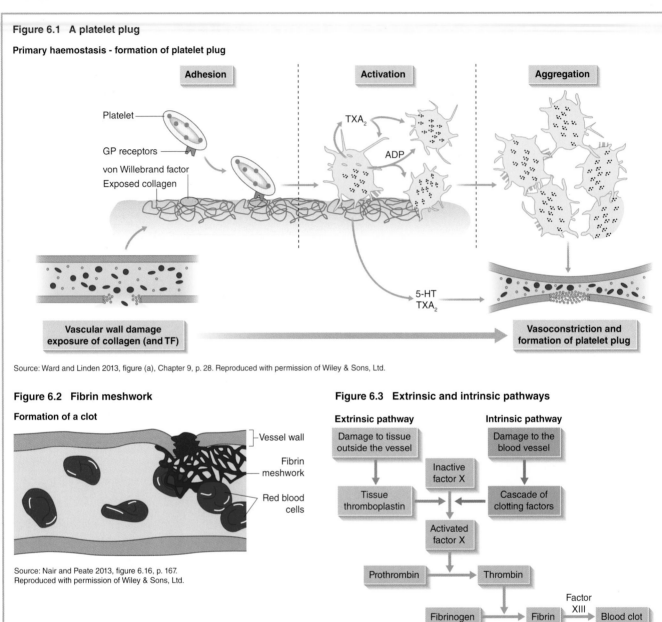

Figure 6.1 A platelet plug

Primary haemostasis - formation of platelet plug

Adhesion

Activation

Aggregation

Platelet

GP receptors

von Willebrand factor
Exposed collagen

TXA$_2$

ADP

5-HT
TXA$_2$

**Vascular wall damage
exposure of collagen (and TF)**

**Vasoconstriction and
formation of platelet plug**

Source: Ward and Linden 2013, figure (a), Chapter 9, p. 28. Reproduced with permission of Wiley & Sons, Ltd.

Figure 6.2 Fibrin meshwork

Formation of a clot

Vessel wall

Fibrin
meshwork

Red blood
cells

Source: Nair and Peate 2013, figure 6.16, p. 167.
Reproduced with permission of Wiley & Sons, Ltd.

Figure 6.3 Extrinsic and intrinsic pathways

Extrinsic pathway

Intrinsic pathway

Damage to tissue
outside the vessel

Damage to the
blood vessel

Inactive
factor X

Tissue
thromboplastin

Cascade of
clotting factors

Activated
factor X

Prothrombin

Thrombin

Fibrinogen

Fibrin

Factor
XIII

Blood clot

Physiology of haemostasis

The haemostatic mechanism is complex and delicately balanced. Haemostasis is one aspect of the wound-healing process. The wound healing process passes though a number of phases, including inflammation, granulation and maturation.

Haemostasis is a process that causes bleeding to stop, keeping blood within a damaged blood vessel; the opposite of haemostasis is haemorrhage, and it is the first stage of wound healing.

The body's initial response to wounding is to control the loss of blood from the area. Following damage to blood vessels and endothelial cells, platelets become sticky and adhere to the wall of the blood vessel and to each other, forming a platelet thrombus. The platelet thrombus acts as a temporary plug that reduces blood flow out of the wound (see Figure 6.1). The platelets also release serotonin and other chemical mediators, which results in a short period of vasoconstriction. Haemostasis is also achieved by the activation of the clotting cascade, initiated by damage to the endothelium.

Platelet function

Platelet function is essential in haemostasis. Platelets are vesicle-like fragments; they are incomplete cells, approximately 2–4 μm in diameter, discoid in shape and arise from larger cells, the megakaryocytes, in the bone marrow. The normal platelet count is approximately $3 \times 1011/L$.

Five events occur when there is injury to a blood vessel:

1 local vasoconstriction
2 adhesion and aggregation of platelets
3 activation of the clotting cascade
4 activation of coagulation inhibitors
5 fibrinolysis.

When damage to a blood vessel occurs, it causes it to constrict through direct action and also indirectly through the release of vasoconstrictors from platelets; these actions play a central role in limiting blood loss. Damage to the endothelial lining of the blood vessel also triggers platelet activity; when this happens the platelets aggregate forming a plug. This activity along with the transient vasoconstriction is generally responsible for the cessation of bleeding. Platelets when activated also liberate a number of vasoconstrictor substances, revealing a phospholipid that is essential for the creation of a blood clot.

Generally, platelets do not adhere to the smooth endothelial lining of the blood vessels. However, when the vasculature is damaged, this exposes the blood to subendothelial collagen and microfibrils. The platelets stick to the collagen in the damaged vessel via glycoproteins (GPs) (von Willebrand factor enhances adhesion) that are located on the surface of the platelets. Activation results in the platelets changing shape along with the production of pseudopodia (these are temporary protrusions) producing thromboxane A_2 (TXA_2) – an enzyme (a lipid with prothrombotic properties) – 5-hydroxytryptamine (5-HT or serotonin) and ADP (adenosine diphosphate) release. Further vasoconstriction occurs caused by TXA_2 and 5-HT; ADP recruits more platelets and they aggregate to each other cross-linking with fibrinogen. A soft plug forms that is held together by fibrinogen molecules that form bridges between adjacent platelets. The aggregated platelets occlude the wound, which eventually stops bleeding. This is an unstable primary plug, a loosely aggregated plug, and has to be consolidated into a more stable plug.

Clotting cascade

The clotting cascade provides this more stable consolidated plug and ultimately results in the conversion of the plasma protein fibrinogen to fibrin, which forms a meshwork providing a seal to the damaged vasculature (see Figure 6.2). The cascade is a sequence of interactions between proteins that cause fibrin depositions at the location of tissue injury and is initiated by its interaction with activated factor VII. See Figure 6.3 for the clotting cascade.

The initial phase (this used to be known as the extrinsic pathway) involves several factors. Tissue factor VII and factor VIIa convert factor X to its active form, factor Xa. Tissue factor VIIa also convers factor IX to its activated form, factor IXa; further generation of factor Xa is inhibited by the tissue factor pathway inhibitor. At this point the amount of factor Xa produced is insufficient to sustain coagulation. Further factor Xa to allow haemostasis to progress to completion can now only be generated by the factor IXa pathway; by this stage though enough thrombin has been generated by the factor Xa to activate factors VIII and V. These both act as potent catalysts. Factor VIIIa increases the capacity of factor IXa to activate factor X to Xa many thousand times. The increased factor Xa produced in this way along with its own cofactor, activated Va, forms a complex that promotes the efficient conversion of prothrombin to thrombin. Thrombin then allows the conversion of fibrinogen to fibrin. The final result of the cascade is the production of fibrin, the biological glue that eventually seals the haemostatic plug ensuring haemostasis. As soon as a small amount of thrombin is formed the clotting process accelerates and provides more and more thrombin in to the wound. At high concentrations this thrombin quickly converts fibrinogen to fibrin on the surface of the platelet aggregate to stabilize the haemostatic plug. Over the course of the subsequent 7–12 days, the process of fibrinolysis dissolves the fibrin in the wound as the site of injury heals and the cell layer in the vessel wall is restored. Scar formation occurs, and within a few weeks the wound is completely healed.

Wound healing

Wound healing is a complex and dynamic process that varies according to the location and type of wound and occurs as a systemic process, which follows in stepwise fashion and involves the stages of haemostasis, inflammation and repair. Generally, from injury to resolution, wounds go through four phases:

1 haemostasis
2 inflammation
3 profliferation
4 remodelling.

As fibrin formation occurs a protective wound scab is formed. Scab formation provides a surface beneath which cell migration and movement of the wound edges can follow. As the inflammatory process develops, this brings nutrients to the area of the wound, removes debris and bacteria and makes available chemical stimuli for wound repair to begin to occur. Repair begins instantaneously after wounding and proceeds quickly through the processes of epithelialization, fibroplasia and capillary proliferation into the healing area. Different tissues possess their own normal rates of growth as the healing process occurs. The ideal rate of healing happens when there are factors present that are advantageous to healing and factors that have the ability to disturb or hinder the healing processes are controlled or absent.

7 Inflammation

Figure 7.1 Causes of the inflammatory response

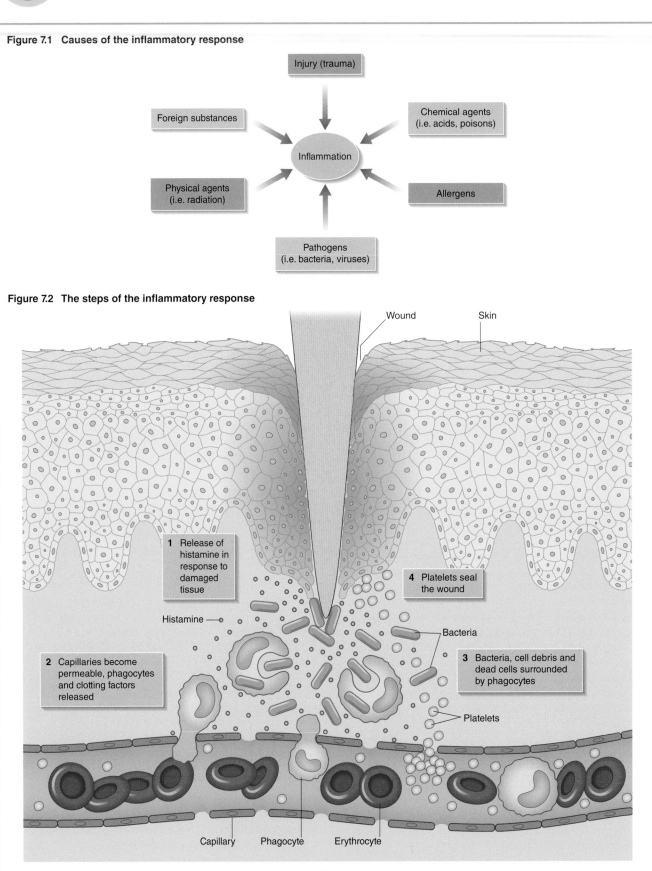

Figure 7.2 The steps of the inflammatory response

Wound   Skin

1 Release of histamine in response to damaged tissue

4 Platelets seal the wound

Histamine

Bacteria

2 Capillaries become permeable, phagocytes and clotting factors released

3 Bacteria, cell debris and dead cells surrounded by phagocytes

Platelets

Capillary   Phagocyte   Erythrocyte

Wound Care at a Glance, First Edition. Ian Peate and Wyn Glencross. © 2015 John Wiley & Sons, Ltd. Published 2015 by John Wiley & Sons, Ltd.
Companion website: www.ataglanceseries.com/nursing/woundcare

Inflammation

When there is insult to the body, for example trauma or intentional injury resulting in damage to the blood vessels the first response is to arrest haemorrhage. Prevention of blood loss and the formation of clots and scabs in an attempt to provide a protective covering when the skin has been broken are part of the haemostatic process.

The body has effective mechanisms to block potential pathogens from entering the body, including the skin and mucous membranes as physical barriers. Enzymes such as lysozyme in tears and sweat have the capacity to destroy many potential pathogens chemically; however, even with these external barriers available to fight potential pathogens, occasions occur when pathogens enter the body. When this occurs and infection is present the body sets into action the inflammatory response. This response is non-specific and attacks any and all foreign invaders. This inflammatory response is a universal reaction to tissue damage. See figure 7.1 for causes of the inflammatory response.

Inflammation attempts to rid the body of microbes, toxins or other foreign material at the site of injury with the intention of preventing their spread to other tissues; it also begins to prepare the site for tissue repair.

The inflammatory response

Inflammation is an innate response to tissue damage, with four phases (or characteristic signs) associated with the inflammatory response:

1 redness (rubor)
2 swelling (tumour)
3 heat (calor)
4 pain (dolor).

Loss of function is a fifth phase added to the original four. Inflammation can result in loss of function; for example, as a result of the inability to detect sensation depending on the site and extent of the injury.

When injury occurs pathogens such as bacteria, virus or fungus gain entry to the body. Almost immediately the damaged cells cause a number of events to happen:

1 vasodilation
2 messenger molecules are released
3 activation of complement
4 extravasation of vascular components
5 phagocytosis
6 pain.

The mast cells injured in the connective tissue release histamine. The arrival of histamine at the site of injury has an immediate impact on blood vessels in the region. Arterioles dilate, venules constrict, causing an increase in blood flow. Vasodilation is brought about by four main mechanisms.

1 The kinin system in the cell produces bradykinin a vasodilator, also responsible for pain.
2 Damaged plasma membranes release arachidonic acid, a fatty acid, a precursor to prostaglandins. Prostaglandins are also vasodilators and have hyperalgesic properties (they increase pain).
3 Release of histamine from the degranulated mast cells increases pore size between the capillary cells, permitting movement of proteins and other micromolecules into interstitial spaces.
4 Vascular epithelial cells release nitric oxide, a vasodilator. Macrophages also release large amounts of nitric oxide.

Increased blood flow explains redness and heat associated with infection. Capillaries within injured tissue dilate, becoming permeable; this is essential for an appropriate inflammatory response, providing an opportunity for some of the blood components to be released into the damaged area and the site of infection (Figure 7.2).

Platelets and clotting factors

Platelets and their associated clotting factors (see Chapter 6) (for example, thrombin and fibrinogen) exit through the leaky capillary walls and migrate towards the site of injury. The clotting factors serve a dual purpose when this occurs, they help to plug the wound and seal damaged blood vessels; they also confine infectious agents to the wound site slowing their systemic spread.

Chemokines

A second line of defence has also been activated. Cells close to the injury release a series of chemical signals radiating from the site of inflammation; these signals are known as chemokines. Concentration of chemokines is greatest immediately surrounding the infection. High levels of chemokines attract or provide a signal for the attraction of phagocytic white blood cells including neutrophils.

Phagocytosis

As chemokine concentration continues to increase, phagocytes leave the capillary entering the site of infection macrophages arrive 24 hours later. Phagocytes engulf and destroy the pathogens present, recognizing the pathogen as non-self matter and send out pseudopodia sounding the pathogen. The wound site begins to heal. After the white blood cells engulf pathogen particles, they begin to die; they eventually make up the pus associated with infected cuts. The key molecule released is interleukin 1, attracting neutrophils and macrophages to the site of injury, helping to clear away debris from the injured area.

Phagocytosis results in a metabolically intensive activity and is responsible for some of the heat associated with inflammation. Pyrexia occurs during infection accompanying inflammation. Bacterial toxins elevate body temperature, releasing cytokines from macrophages causing temperature increase. The presence of pyrexia exaggerates the impact of interferons, hindering the growth of some microbes speeding up reactions that aid repair.

With the pathogen particles destroyed and damaged tissue repaired, histamine signals fade, and blood vessels return to normal size.

Pain is generated by action and interaction of bradykinin and prostaglandins, increasing the sensation of pain in inflammation. Other chemicals are also involved in the stimulation of pain after injury has occurred; lactic acid produced by anaerobic cellular respiration is one example. Hydrogen ions and potassium released from damaged cells also stimulate the pain receptors.

Inflammation lasts for approximately 4–5 days. The process requires energy and nutritional resources for efficacy. With large complex wounds demands made on the body are considerable. Inflammation has a protective function helping to eliminate the cause(s) of tissue damage. Extending the inflammatory stage, for example where there is infection, the presence of a foreign body or damage that has been caused by an inappropriate dressing, can have an adverse effect on the person's health and wellbeing.

Proliferation (granulation and epithelialization)

8

Figure 8.1 Wound-healing time scales

Coagulation		Inflammation	
Vasoconstriction	Polymorphonuclear neutrophils predominant		Macrophages predominant
	Vasodilation	Fibroblast proliferation and migration	Angiogenesis
		Fibroplasia and granulation tissue formation	50% of normal tissue strength
			Collagen deposition	Maturation and remodeling

Phases of wound healing
- Limit is within faded interval
- Limit is not defined

Epithelialization
- incomplete basement membrane
- complete basement membrane

Contraction

1	2 3 4 5	10	20 30	1	2	3 4 5 6	12	1	2	3 4 5 6 1	2	3	1	2	3 4 5 6	1	2 3
minutes				60	hours			24	48	days 7	14	weeks	7 10	months		12	years

Figure 8.2 Proliferative phase of wound healing showing fibroblasts producing extracellular matrix and re-epithelialization by keratinocytes

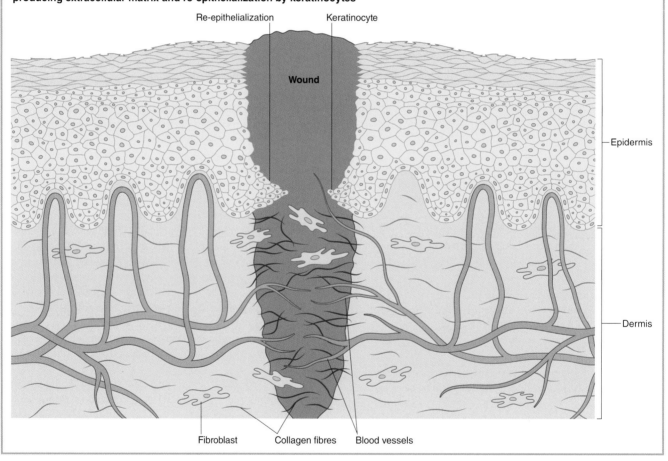

Re-epithelialization   Keratinocyte

Wound

Epidermis

Dermis

Fibroblast   Collagen fibres   Blood vessels

Wound Care at a Glance, First Edition. Ian Peate and Wyn Glencross. © 2015 John Wiley & Sons, Ltd. Published 2015 by John Wiley & Sons, Ltd.
Companion website: www.ataglanceseries.com/nursing/woundcare

Wound healing consists of filling the gap created by tissue destruction followed by restoration of the structural continuity of the injured part through three phases of healing (Figure 8.1):

1 the inflammatory phase
2 the proliferative phase
3 the remodelling phase.

Proliferation

The proliferation phase overlaps with the inflammation stage (see Chapter 7) as this phase starts to end. The focus of the proliferative phase is associated with the building of new tissue to fill the wound space. As the inflammation diminishes, work begins to repair the injury. About 3 days after injury, fibroblasts will have started to enter and assemble in the wound; this is the start of the transition from inflammatory phase to proliferation phase. The fibroblasts are connective tissue cells that synthesize and secrete collagen as well as the secretion of growth factors that induce the growth of blood vessels through the process of angiogenesis and at the same time promoting endothelial cell proliferation and migration. As the fibroblasts grow and form they produce a new, provisional extracellular matrix that has come about by excreting collagen and fibronectin.

The fibroblasts and endothelial cells form granulation tissue that acts as the foundation for scar tissue development (Figure 8.2).

Granulation

Granulation tissue contains newly developed capillary buds. Granulation tissue can now be seen in the wound around the end of the first week; this tissue continues to grow until the wound has healed. This tissue is rich in new blood vessels and other components that are required to fill in the injured tissue. Granulation tissue is usually bright red or pink, moist, soft to the touch and has a bumpy appearance. Granulation tissue is fragile and bleeds easily. The masses within the injured tissue keep growing and contracting depending on the wound type; this takes approximately 8 weeks for a standard open healing excision wound and 4 weeks for a closed (sutured) wound.

Around day 5 post injury, exudate appears in the wound (this is the by-product of healing and is a sticky greenish-white substance resembling pus but is not). If too much exudate is produced, wound healing may be slowed; increased exudate may be an indication of infection and increased oedema.

Epithelialization, maturation and remodelling

The final feature of the proliferative stage is epithelialization, this is the regeneration, migration, proliferation and differentiation of epithelial cells at the wound's edge form a new surface area similar to that destroyed by the injury. As soon as injury has occurred, cytokines are released from platelets and they activate keratinocytes. As the migration of keratinocytes occurs, re-epithelialization begins as early as 2 hours after wounding. Growth factors such as keratinocytes growth factor (KGF) and epidermal growth factor (EGF) provoke proliferation and migration of keratinocytes.

The main sources of migrating keratinocytes during re-epithelialization process are basal keratinocytes from the wound edges, dermal appendages such as hair follicles, sweat glands and sebaceous glands, and bone marrow-derived keratinocyte stem cells. Keratinocytes secrete proteases and plasminogen activator that activates plasmin. Migration of keratinocytes over the wound site is also enhanced by lack of contact inhibition and release of nitric oxide from polymorphonuclear leucocytes (PMNs), keratinocytes and fibroblasts. Epithelial cells continue migrating across the wound bed until cells from different sides meet in the middle, at this point contact between keratinocytes inhibits further migration. New layers of keratinocytes differentiate and this gives rise to a stratified epidermis.

As the proliferative stage ends white bloods cells leave the area and oedema diminishes and the wound begins to blanch as the small blood vessels begin to thrombose and degenerate.

The maturation and remodelling phases overlap with the proliferation phase as healing begins to come to an end. The remodelling phase begins after about 3 weeks and can continue for 6 months or longer. Final scar tissue starts to form by the simultaneous synthesis of lysis and collagen. Collagen is fibrous in character, connects and supports tissues and organs such as skin, bone, tendons, muscles and cartilage. It is often referred to as the glue that holds the body together; it is collagen that provides tensile strength. There are over 25 types of collagens that occur naturally in the body; it can be found both inside and outside cells, contributing to the structure of cells.

At this stage the process of remodelling of the collagen fibres is laid down. The scar becomes avascular.

The wound is made smaller by the action of myofibroblasts; as the edges of the wound are drawn closer together this establishes a grip on the edges of the wound, causing them to contract using a mechanism that is similar to that in smooth muscle cells. When the role of myofibroblasts is close to completion, cells that are no longer needed undergo apoptosis. Myofibroblastic activity can persist, contributing to fibrosis and scarring in the skin.

Nerve endings are now redeveloping and the tissue is starting to rearrange itself. Scar tissue may achieve 70–80% of tensile strength by the end of 3 months. Within the tissue there is much physiological activity still occurring after surface wound healing has occurred. This final phase continues for up to 18 months after the wound has closed.

Rapid keratinocyte migration along with re-epithelialization can often lead to better wound-healing outcomes and decreased scar formation. However, exposure to air and/or lack of moisture will result in a delay in the healing process.

This whole process is complex and the skin is fragile and prone to interruption or failure and the outcome of this is the formation of non-healing chronic wounds. There are factors that may contribute to interruption or failure and these include:

- diabetes
- venous or arterial disease
- infection
- ageing.

Maturation

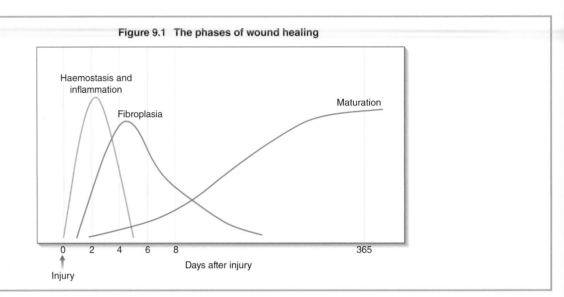

Figure 9.1 The phases of wound healing

Wound healing

This text has explained that there are many factors associated with the healing of wounds, for example, internal (coexisting disease, the ageing process, nutritional status and external (pressure, friction, sheer) factors. Wound healing is a natural response to tissue injury, a restorative response. When healing occurs this is as the result of the interaction of a complex cascade of cellular events that produces resurfacing, reconstitution and restoration of the tensile strength of the skin that has been injured. There are also a number of phases of wound healing (Figure 9.1):

- the vascular response (this is where haemostasis takes place)
- the inflammatory response (here the body puts in place a variety of inflammatory responses)
- the proliferation phase (the active growth phase with granulation and epithelisation occurring)
- the maturation phase.

While healing is a systematic process the four classic phases noted above overlap, often (as is the case here) and for the sake of discussion and understanding, the process of wound healing is usually presented as a series of separate discrete events. In reality it must be noted that the whole process is much more complicated, as cellular events that lead to scar formation overlap. There are many aspects of wound healing that are still to be understood.

The maturation phase

Collagen

During the maturation phase collagen remodelling depends on continued collagen synthesis in the presence of collagen destruction. In the wound collagenases and matrix metalloproteinases (an enzyme) helps with the removal of excess collagen as the synthesis of new collagen persists. Tissue inhibitors of metalloproteinases limit these collagenolytic enzymes, helping ensure that a balance exists between creation of new collagen and elimination of old collagen.

As remodelling occurs, collagen becomes more organized. A number of complex interactions take place with fibronectin gradually disappearing and hyaluronic acid and glycosaminoglycans replaced by proteoglycans. The types of collagen change and type III collagen is replaced by type I collagen. Water is resorbed from the scar. When these events occur this allows the collagen fibres to lie closer together, enabling collagen cross-linking and ultimately reducing scar thickness. Intramolecular and intermolecular collagen cross-links result in increased wound bursting strength (tensile strength). Approximately 21 days after injury, when the net collagen content of the wound is stable remodelling begins, this can continue indefinitely.

The measurement of the tensile strength of a wound is its load capacity per unit area. The bursting strength of a wound is associated with the force needed to break a wound regardless of its dimension. Bursting strength differs according to skin thickness. Following approximately 60 days after injury peak tensile strength of the wound occurs. When the wound heals it will only reach approximately 80% of the tensile strength of unwounded skin.

Cytokines

These are significant mediators of wound healing events. A cytokine is a protein mediator that is released from numerous cell sources, binding to cell surface receptors with the purpose of stimulating a cell response.

Cytokines can reach their target cell via various routes. The first cytokine described was epidermal growth factor, which is a potent mitogen (a substance that encourages cell division) for epithelial cells, endothelial cells and fibroblasts. Epidermal growth factor stimulates other activity in the wound healing factors fibronectin synthesis, angiogenesis, fibroplasia, and collagenase activity. Fibroblast growth factor stimulates for angiogenesis. This factor also stimulates wound contraction and epithelialization and production of collagen.

Platelet derivative growth factor (PDGF) is released from the platelets and is responsible for the stimulation of neutrophils and macrophages and is a mitogen and chemotactic agent for fibroblasts and smooth muscle cells stimulating angiogenesis, collagen synthesis, and collagenase.

Transforming growth factor-β is an important stimulant for fibroblast proliferation and the production of proteoglycans, collagen, and fibrin. The factor promotes accumulation of the extracellular matrix and fibrosis; it has the ability to reduce scarring and to reverse the inhibition of wound healing.

Tumour necrosis factor-α is produced by macrophages and stimulates angiogenesis and the synthesis of collagen and collagenase. This factor is a mitogen for fibroblasts.

During the maturation phase (also known as the reconstruction phase)remodelling of the scar continues for approximately 1 year. Scar tissue regains about two thirds of its original strength, it will never be as strong as the original tissue it replaces. Maturation is the final phase occurring once the wound has closed. This phase includes the remodelling of collagen from type III to type I. Cellular activity reduces and the number of blood vessels in the wounded area regress and decrease.

The ability to closely approximate uninjured tissue is very much dependent on size, depth, location and type of wound, as well as the person's nutritional status, wound care and the individual's overall health.

10 Factors affecting wound healing

Figure 10.1 Holistic assessment

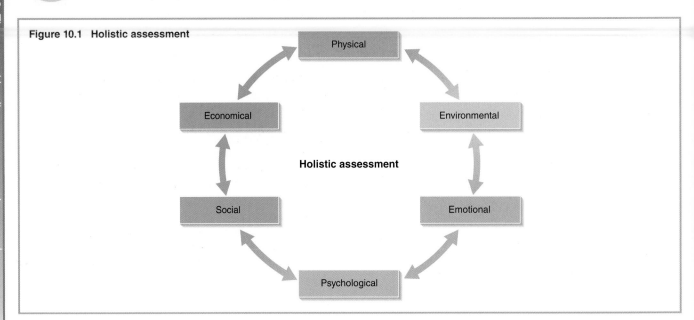

Holistic assessment

There are many factors that influence the healing process and healing rates of wounds; these include physical, environmental, emotional, psychological, and social and economical factors. In order to ensure a wound progresses, as far as is possible, through the normal healing process, within a reasonable time frame, it is crucial that these aspects are considered when carrying out a wound assessment. Simply assessing the wound in isolation will not identify any issues that may be preventing a wound from healing, or which could be slowing down the rate at which it will heal. Therefore a holistic assessment must be completed as regularly as a wound assessment in order to identify and rectify any potential delays in the wound healing rates. The holistic and wound assessment process will be discussed later in Chapter 17, and, in the meantime, Figure 10.1 shows how each factor can impact on each other. Let us briefly consider some of these factors and how they can affect the patient and healing rates.

Physical

This factor considers the patient in the physical sense, for example age, gender, underlying medical conditions, medications, physique; weight, height and lifestyle. In other words, all intrinsic factors associated with the patient. Failure to identify and address relevant physical issues, where it is possible to address them, could not only impact on the wounds' ability to heal but also on the following holistic issues.

Many aspects of the patient can't be altered such as age; however, certain medical conditions, although perhaps incurable, could be controlled to optimize the patient's health and healing prospects, such as diabetes.

Environmental

External factors can impact on a wound's ability to heal; therefore consideration must be given to this aspect when assessing the patient, for example the environment the patient is nursed in; it is important to consider who (if anyone) is providing care to the patient: is the care appropriate, are the staff/carers knowledgeable about standards of care? Is the patient's clothing or footwear appropriate and not ill fitting? Ill-fitting items could reduce circulation or add pressure to the patient's skin, resulting in wound deterioration or pressure damage. What about the surface the patient is sitting or lying on? What about medical devices? Surfaces and devices can easily cause pressure damage or affect the circulation to a wound if these things are in the same vicinity. Has the patient got access to good nutrition? Who is providing the food, what quality of food is it? The environment as a whole must be considered when assessing the patient (more on this later).

The wound environment must be considered, as this could be an issue if an inappropriate dressing is applied that does not maintain a moist wound-healing environment that is conducive to optimum healing, or if the wound dressings are being tampered with by the patient or others (such as family, carers and other untrained, unskilled persons).

Emotional

What is affecting the patient's feelings: are they worried about income? Do they have family worries or stressors? Do they have pain of any sort or anything else that could affect their emotions such as bereavement or loneliness? Emotional issues is known to impact on the patient's physical well-being and skin integrity, and this can be evidenced in some people who are prone to developing rashes or herpes simplex (cold sores) when under a lot of emotional strain.

Psychological

This factor can be linked quite closely with the symptoms resulting from emotions that can impact on the patient's psychological status, which could lead to psychological breakdown. It is important to consider such things as mental illness, neurological impairments such as dementia, all of which could affect the patient's mental capacity (either permanent or temporary). Psychological issues can impact on the patient's physical wellbeing in a similar way to any emotional burdens they may have, whilst exacerbating those emotions.

Social

Examples of social issues could be loneliness and isolation, poor housing and/or living conditions, poor nutrition, poor standards in hygiene, overcrowding and lifestyle. This factor also can be linked to emotional and psychological status of a patient, and if left unaddressed could impact on the physical wellbeing of the patient. For example, a patient with a malodorous wound could become isolated due to embarrassment about the odour omitting from their wound. In time the patient could become housebound, lose their independence and become lonely due to the lack of socialising.

Economical

This factor could identify financial issues with the patient that for example could impact on the type and quality of nutrition the patient is able to afford; it could be due to a cost issue with regards to lack of appropriate bedding, seating, clothing or footwear all of which could impact on the patient's wound and skin integrity as a whole. This factor could also impact on all of the aforementioned factors, particularly with regard to socioeconomics.

We must also consider the type of dressing we are selecting for use on their wounds; whilst we must always aim for cost-effectiveness, it is not always the cheapest or most expensive product that is most appropriate.

While cost must be a consideration in all of the above economical aspects, much of it will be out of our control and will be dependent on the patient's own budget. However, where possible, we must give due consideration to the patient's needs and, it must not be the main driving force when selecting any products, devices.

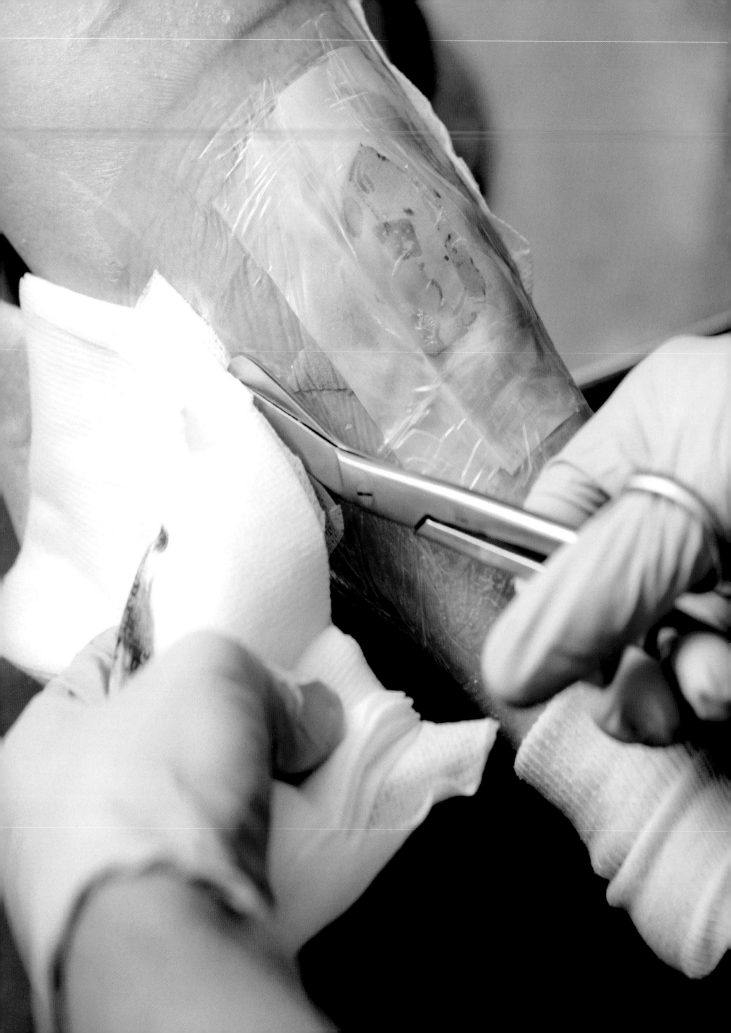

The abnormal healing process: chronic wound healing

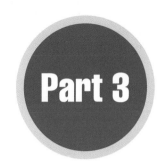

Part 3

Chapters

 Visit the companion website at **www.ataglanceseries.com/nursing/woundcare** to test yourself on these topics.

The impaired healing process

Factors that affect the healing process can be intrinsic (i.e. related to the persons physical make up), extrinsic (i.e. external to the person) or both (i.e. intrinsic and extrinsic). Let us now look at these factors and consider how they can hinder the normal process that we have already discussed, and consider how these can be managed in order to prompt a wound to progress through the normal phases of wound healing within a reasonable timescale as stated in the previous chapter.

Considering both intrinsic and extrinsic factors let us look at the four phases of wound healing and the potential factors that could affect that process:

1 Haemostasis: The wound does not stop bleeding within 5–10 minutes, even though pressure has been applied. The cause of continued bleeding may be due to a severed large blood vessel; a clotting disorder such as low platelets or haemophilia; or the patient may be taking anticoagulant medications such as aspirin or warfarin. If the wound does not reach haemostasis (with firm pressure) within 10–20 minutes the patient will require immediate medical assistance.

2 Inflammatory response: There are two potential ways that this response can be interrupted.

(a) A wound may not enter this phase due to the patient taking anti-inflammatory medication (which stops the increase in the blood supply to the wound bed); or they may have a severely reduced blood supply whereby white blood cells (e.g. phagocytes) do not reach the site of the injury. In either event the wound will either progress slowly or not at all through this phase during which time the wound is at great risk of infection due to the lack of essential white cells reaching the wound bed.

(b) A patient may have an inflammatory condition such as rheumatoid arthritis, ulcerative colitis or Crohn's disease and if their condition is in 'flare-up' when they develop a wound, then it is probable that the wound will enter this phase but will remain in this phase. This means that the wound is unable to progress to healing and over time will be vulnerable to infection as bacterial levels on the wound bed increase over time (discussed in later chapters).

3 Regenerative phase: This is the most common phase for delays in wound healing and is usually due to an extrinsic factor, such as incorrect dressing choices, poor dressing technique and poor exudate management. For example, if a dressing is allowed to adhere to a wound, it will cause trauma to the wound bed on dressing removal and so the wound has to once again go through the inflammatory response, thereby delaying wound healing by up to 5 days. Similarly, if a dressing is allowed to become saturated, migrating granulation and epithelial cells will become macerated and will be destroyed, so healing is unable to take place. The longer a wound takes to heal the more likely it will become infected as the bio-burden increases on the wound bed over time.

4 Maturation phase: This is the 'shrinking' phase of wound healing whereby the collagen and elastic fibre matrix reorganizes in order to increase the tensile strength of the scar tissue. This process continues throughout the healing process in symmetry with the regenerative phase, and continues for many years after the wound has completely re-epithelialized.

As the tissues shrink, contractures can occur, particularly over the palm of hands, face and joints, which can restrict movement. Occasionally keloid and hypertrophic scaring can occur, with poor cosmetic results. Often massage can reduce these effects of abnormal maturation of tissues by assisting with the redistribution of collagen and elastic fibres. Occasionally plastic surgeons recommend the use of Silicone creams and dressings to reduce the effects of scarring and contractures, however the evidence behind the efficacy of these products are limited to date.

While some of the factors that hinder the healing rates of a given individual are uncontrollable, others are not, and it is therefore essential that the nurse responsible for assessing, treating and managing a wound carries out a holistic assessment that considers both extrinsic and intrinsic factors before deciding on the most appropriate management for any given wound. This is rather like a doctor prescribing a drug; they ensure that they are fully aware of the comorbidities and medication before prescribing something new. The formal assessment process must therefore consider the following before treating the wound:

1 Extrinsic factors (this list is not exhaustive)
Clothing, footwear, bed, chair, home environment, lifestyle, dressing choice, nurse/carer knowledge and expertise in wound management, patient knowledge and compliance, nutrition, socioeconomic status.

2 Intrinsic factors (this list is not exhaustive)
Age, gender, comorbidities, allergies, medications, skin type, scarring, nutrition, incontinence and immobility.

3 Finally, the wound assessment must consider
Dimensions, depth, peri-wound skin condition, exudate levels, tissue type, signs of infection (to be discussed later).

Wound Care at a Glance, First Edition. Ian Peate and Wyn Glencross. © 2015 John Wiley & Sons, Ltd. Published 2015 by John Wiley & Sons, Ltd.
Companion website: www.ataglanceseries.com/nursing/woundcare

12 Factors affecting wound healing

There are many reasons why wounds do not heal in a straight-forward manner; these reasons can be classified as intrinsic (something internal to the individual) or extrinsic (something external to the individual). On occasions factors may be both intrinsic as well as extrinsic as this chapter will explain. It is vital that the patient is assessed holistically so that influencing factors of delayed healing rates can be identified and addressed as far as possible, after which the wound itself can be assessed. Below are some common factors that impact on wound healing rates and should be considered during assessments. Many of the factors mentioned below have been discussed in greater detail in other chapters:

Intrinsic factors

Age – as we age cell regeneration rates slow down, which means that wounds usually take longer to heal the older we get. A wound that might take 3 weeks to heal in a youth may take 6 weeks to heal in the older individual. It is therefore important to set realistic goals when planning care.

Gender – the fluctuating hormone levels in females during their lifetime appear to affect skin integrity and therefore healing rates, albeit in a mild way.

Psychological – it is thought that the psychological state can impact on wound healing, such as high levels of emotional stress, worry and negative thought processes. Evidence of this can be seen where a person develops mouth ulcer or cold sores when they are experiencing such emotional pressures.

Physical/structure – the human form itself can be a factor in wound healing rates, and one example of this is where pressure ulcers exist; the underlying bone that caused the ulcer in the first instance will continue to delay wound healing if pressure relief is not ensured. Other physical factors that must be considered are for example scar tissue, physical deformities, particularly of limbs, amputations, mobility and reduced mobility.

Lifestyle – smoking, alcohol and drug use, although an extrinsic factor, can impact intrinsically on the individual, which could delay healing rates.

Nutrition – this can be both an intrinsic factor (e.g. due to malabsorption conditions or gastric surgery) and an extrinsic factor (due to dietary choices) all of which can result in poor nutritional intake. As wounds require an increased nutritional intake, any reduction will impact on healing rates.

Medications – common medications that impact on wound healing processes and rates are steroids, anti-inflammatory and cytotoxic drugs.

Comorbidities – common medical conditions that affect wound healing rates are:

- Diabetes, peripheral artery disease and other conditions that affect the blood circulation such as heart disease and hypertension means a reduced blood supply reaches the wound bed.
- An inefficient cardiopulmonary circulation due to heart or lung disease means that the wound will receive a reduced supply of essential oxygen and nutrients that will reduce healing rates.
- Inflammatory diseases, such as rheumatoid arthritis and ulcerative colitis; these conditions affect the inflammatory phase of a wound healing if the condition is in 'flare-up', which can cause a prolonged inflammatory phase; alternatively if the condition is in remission the patient is usually taking prescribed steroids, which also delay the healing process by delaying or stopping the inflammatory phase. Patients on steroids who are due to have surgery are often required to stop steroids for a short time before and after surgery.
- Cancer.
- Major or multi-organ failure.

Extrinsic factors

Environment – this may include the surface the patient is lying or sitting on; the environment they live in; the support networks available to the patient; social and financial factors. It can also refer to the environment the wound is kept in (see below).

Wound dressing – an inappropriate dressing that maintains an adverse wound environment (e.g. too wet) can cause trauma and/or delayed healing.

Clothing and footwear – these can impact on healing rates by causing pressure or restriction of blood supply, which means that there is a reduce supply of essential oxygen and nutrients supplied to the wound.

Wound site – wounds sited over joints (e.g. elbows, knees) will usually take slightly longer to heal than wounds over non-mobile areas.

Temperature – of particular importance is the temperature of the wound bed; ideally a wound ought to be retained at body temperature (i.e. 36.9°C). If the wound is not dressed with an appropriate (insulating) dressing the wound bed will cool according to the atmosphere and will result in a reduced blood supply. The temperature of an individual is also important; if a person is allowed to cool the peripheral circulation will be reduced in order to preserve the core temperature. This in turn reduces the amount of blood (and therefore oxygen and nutrients) reaching the wound bed.

Nutrition – it is vital that the patient with a wound takes in additional calories in order to increase healing rates, particularly with regards to increased proteins.

Wound care skill/technique – one of the most common reasons for delayed wound healing is the wound care technique of health professionals. This may include the use of inappropriate dressings, causing trauma on removal of the dressing (causing the wound to revert back to the beginning of the healing process); leaving a dressing *in situ* for too long, causing saturation and subsequent maceration/excoriation of the wound and peri-wound tissues.

The list above is not exhaustive and many unique factors not listed here may apply to individuals, such as a rare medical condition or a particular lifestyle. In order to ensure all potential factors that relate to any individual are identified, it is vital that a holistic assessment is completed at the onset of the wound and regularly throughout the healing process in order to identify all factors that may or may not be managed, so that delayed wound healing times can be avoided.

13 Nutrition and wound healing

Figure 13.1 Malnutrition universal screening tool

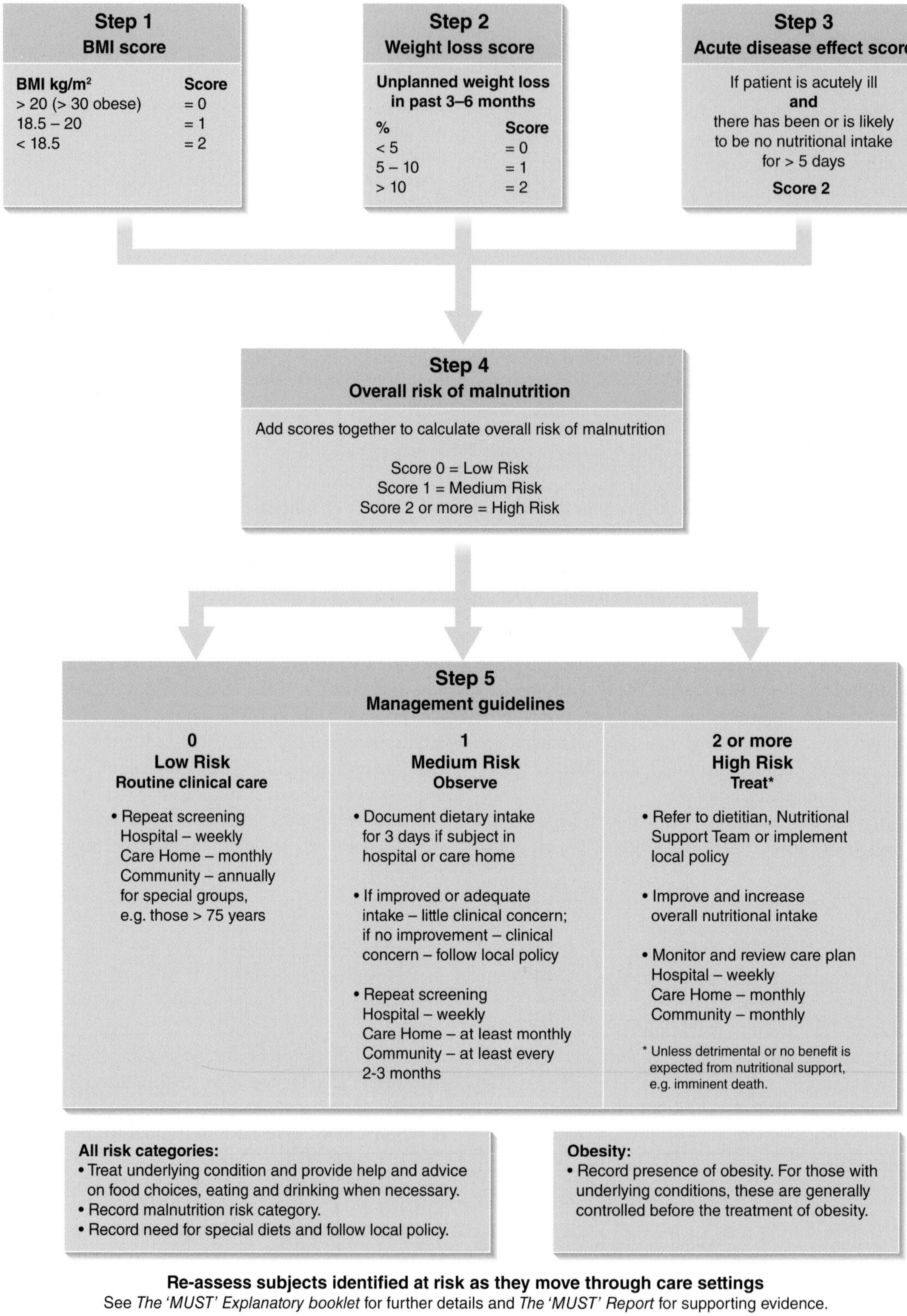

Step 1
BMI score
BMI kg/m² Score
> 20 (> 30 obese) = 0
18.5 – 20 = 1
< 18.5 = 2
Step 2
Weight loss score
Unplanned weight loss in past 3–6 months
% Score
< 5 = 0
5 – 10 = 1
> 10 = 2
Step 3
Acute disease effect score
If patient is acutely ill and there has been or is likely to be no nutritional intake for > 5 days
Score 2
Step 4
Overall risk of malnutrition
Add scores together to calculate overall risk of malnutrition
Score 0 = Low Risk
Score 1 = Medium Risk
Score 2 or more = High Risk
Step 5
Management guidelines
0
Low Risk
Routine clinical care
• Repeat screening
Hospital – weekly
Care Home – monthly
Community – annually for special groups, e.g. those > 75 years
1
Medium Risk
Observe
• Document dietary intake for 3 days if subject in hospital or care home
• If improved or adequate intake – little clinical concern; if no improvement – clinical concern – follow local policy
• Repeat screening
Hospital – weekly
Care Home – at least monthly
Community – at least every 2-3 months
2 or more
High Risk
Treat*
• Refer to dietitian, Nutritional Support Team or implement local policy
• Improve and increase overall nutritional intake
• Monitor and review care plan
Hospital – weekly
Care Home – monthly
Community – monthly
* Unless detrimental or no benefit is expected from nutritional support, e.g. imminent death.
All risk categories:
• Treat underlying condition and provide help and advice on food choices, eating and drinking when necessary.
• Record malnutrition risk category.
• Record need for special diets and follow local policy.
Obesity:
• Record presence of obesity. For those with underlying conditions, these are generally controlled before the treatment of obesity.
Re-assess subjects identified at risk as they move through care settings
See The 'MUST' Explanatory booklet for further details and The 'MUST' Report for supporting evidence.

Source: The Malnutrition Advisory Group 2004, figure on p. 3. Reproduced with permission of BAPEN.

Wound Care at a Glance, First Edition. Ian Peate and Wyn Glencross. © 2015 John Wiley & Sons, Ltd. Published 2015 by John Wiley & Sons, Ltd.
Companion website: www.ataglanceseries.com/nursing/woundcare

Good nutrition is essential for wound healing. A person's nutritional status is a good indicator of the individual's ability to heal as malnutrition can significantly impair all aspects and phases of wound healing leading to delayed healing times. The longer a wound takes to heal the more likely it is to become infected or become complex in nature.

Although many patients with a poor nutritional status develop non-complicated wounds that go on to heal without any attention to their diet, many patients with chronic and/or complex wounds and/or conditions will require thorough assessment and attention to their nutritional intake to optimize healing rates.

A good diet will consist of nutrients that will include protein, carbohydrates, fat, water, vitamins and minerals, as each have a part to play in each of the four phases of wound healing discussed in earlier chapters. Let us briefly consider each of these products and see how they relate to the healing process.

Proteins – contain amino acids that are the building blocks of protein, which is essential for tissue repair and regeneration. A deficiency in protein will significantly impair collagen synthesis, granulation tissue formation and angiogenesis, and the maturation phases of wound healing.

Carbohydrates – provide the energy in the form of glucose needed to power the repair and regeneration process described above.

Fats – are essential in providing an energy source when the carbohydrate sources have been depleted. It is also required to help with thermoregulation (insulation) and it carries fat-soluble vitamins A, E and K, required for wound healing.

Water – A dehydrated patient will lead to a dehydrated wound. A dehydrated wound will delay wound healing as the migration of granulation tissue across the wound bed depends on a fluid environment, which also aids cell functioning. Additionally, wounds will drain fluid (exudate) and if the wound surface area is large or the wound is heavily exuding the patient will require an increased fluid intake over and above the normal requirement of 40–60 mL of water per kilogram of body weight per day, in order to prevent dehydration.

Vitamins (A, C, K, B complex, E) – **Vitamin A** is essential for healthy skin and epithelial integrity; it promotes granulation, angiogenesis and epithelial tissue formation. **Vitamin C** is essential for building and maintaining healthy tissues and it assists the body in absorbing iron. **Vitamin K** is essential for blood clotting, thereby allowing the wound to progress through the inflammatory response and beyond. **B complex vitamins** are a group of eight vitamins required for normal immune functioning and energy metabolism. They aid in white blood cell function and resistance to infection, while improving the tensile strength of the wound. **Vitamin E** is an antioxidant that helps prevent cellular damage; it decreases the inflammatory phase of wound healing; it enhances immune function and decreases platelet adhesion.

Minerals (zinc, iron, copper and magnesium, calcium and phosphorus) – all are important to the wound healing process; **zinc** is an antioxidant vital to cell processes and normal immune function; **iron** is an essential part of haemoglobin and is required for oxygen transportation to cells to maintain life; **copper** is required for haemoglobin synthesis and iron absorption and transportation and increases the strength of collagen fibres; **magnesium** is essential to all living cells and plays an important role in the transportation of calcium and ions across cell membranes, important for muscle contraction, nerve impulse conduction and normal cardiac rhythm; **calcium** is essential for bone formation, remodelling and muscle contraction, for fibrin syntheses and blood clotting; **phosphorus** is essential for normal metabolism and is an essential component of many enzyme systems.

Nutritional assessment

A malnourished and/or dehydrated patient will be at greater risk of wound complications such as wound dehiscence (primary intention), delayed healing rates, wound infection, sepsis and even death. It is therefore essential that routine assessments and reassessments, including weight measurements, are carried out on a patient with a wound in order to ensure that they are receiving an optimum diet and fluids that is sufficient for their wound healing requirements. A nutritional risk assessment tool must be used in order to assist the practitioner in establishing a risk level, but this must not be used in isolation and the practitioner should therefore not replace clinical judgement. Figure 10.1 demonstrates the Malnutrition Universal Screening Tool (MUST) recommended for use by the National Institute of Clinical Excellence. This is a simple to use tool that will give an indication of the patient's risk of malnutrition. A more in depth assessment and referral will be necessary if the patient is deemed to be at risk or if any of the following clinical characteristics as noted.

Clinical characteristics of malnutrition

The clinical characteristics of malnutrition and dehydration that the practitioner must be aware of are emaciation, obesity, transparent skin, pallor, broken blood vessels in the skin, pale eye membranes, missing teeth or poor dentition, bleeding gums, mouth sores and recent changes in body weight (increase or decrease).

Clinical characteristics of the wound caused by malnutrition

In cases where the patient is poorly nourished the wound may present with stagnant or prolonged healing rates including chronic wounds, repeat ulcerations, pressure ulcer formation, neuropathic ulcer formation and friable tissue on the wound bed (fragile and bleeds easily).

Medical conditions that could lead to malnutrition

There are many medical conditions that make it more probable that the patient will develop malnutrition and the practitioner must be extra vigilant in the following examples:

Diabetes mellitus; intestinal conditions; malabsorption conditions (e.g. coeliac disease); cancer; HIV/AIDS; obesity, dysphagia and any patient receiving parental nutrition.

14 Incontinence and wounds

Figure 14.1   An incontinence lesion

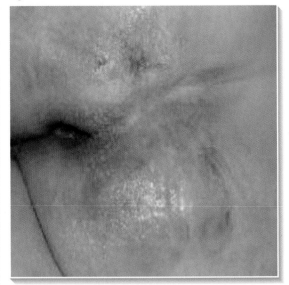

Figure 14.2   Pressure damage exacerbated by moisture lesions

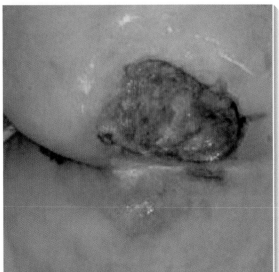

Table 14.1   Features of pressure ulcers and moisture lesions

Pressure ulcer	Moisture lesion
Usually occurs over a bony prominence such as over the sacrum, or under anything that applies constant pressure to the skin, e.g. under the tight elastic on underwear	Occurs where there is excess moisture against the skin. The area may be extensive and over areas where there are no bones immediately underneath the skin, e.g. the buttocks, groins
Usually round in shape to begin with and confined to the area directly over the bone	Appears initially as a rash or a tiny graze(s) that is sporadic over the area of moisture
The onset of pressure damage appears red (when it is a Grade 1). When pressed it is non-blanching (this is when it remains red when pressed)	Appears red, and when pressed the red area blanches (i.e. it goes white)
The skin surrounding the ulcer is usually dry	The skin around the lesions appears 'wet'
The depth of damage can go deep down to muscle, bones and tendons	Is usually superficial, although if pressure is applied on these areas, the damage can go deep as with pressure ulcers. These ulcers will be categorised as pressure ulcers, with a moisture lesion onset
Can become infected, although this is unusual with good wound management. Therefore any infection will be delayed, if at all	Can usually become infected very quickly due to the presence of bodily fluids and matter that harbours bacterial growth
Usually hot or lumpy to touch	Usually cool to touch, unless infected
The patient complains of pain	The patient usually complains of a stinging sensation

Wound Care at a Glance, First Edition. Ian Peate and Wyn Glencross. © 2015 John Wiley & Sons, Ltd. Published 2015 by John Wiley & Sons, Ltd.
Companion website: www.ataglanceseries.com/nursing/woundcare

What is incontinence?

Incontinence is the inability to control bladder and/or bowel functions. It affects people of all ages; however, females are twice as likely as men to develop incontinence. When such a problem exists it can impact not only on the quality of the individual's life and ones dignity, but on the quality of the skin unless adequate steps are taken to prevent moisture damage.

The affects of incontinence

The moisture from urine and faeces can cause maceration (i.e. water logging) of the skin and presents as white soggy area of skin; however, due to the acidic nature of bodily fluids, this moisture can also cause excoriation (burning) of the skin, which presents as a red, wet skin (see Figure 14.1).

Once the skin is macerated and/or excoriated this will result in the loss of the protective layer (via the cuboids cells) and will therefore make the affected area much more vulnerable to bacterial invasion; bacteria will multiply in the moisture and the faecal matter and could result in skin infections (cellulitis).

Once maceration and/or excoriation have occurred, the area will also be much more vulnerable to the effects of pressure, thereby increasing the likelihood and speed at which a pressure ulcer will develop if adequate pressure ulcer prevention and continence care is not provided.

Many people with urinary incontinence will restrict their fluid intake believing this will better control the problem. Unfortunately this will inevitably lead to dehydrated skin, which will be weaker than it would be if it was well hydrated and so will experience damage easier than it would do otherwise. Additionally, a dry skin will absorb moisture from incontinence (and sweating often associated with infection) and will become macerated or excoriated easier than if it was not dehydrated. Furthermore, dehydration can also lead to urinary tract infections, which in turn result in worsened urinary incontinence (and sweating) thereby resulting in increased risk of moisture damage.

Moisture lesion or a pressure ulcer?

Very often moisture lesions are mistaken for pressure ulcers, particularly early-onset pressure ulcers (i.e. Grades 1 or 2), as they can look very similar in appearance. Figure 14.2 demonstrates a Grade 4 pressure ulcer that originated from a moisture lesion. You can see the continued affects of moisture on the skin surrounding the ulcer due to the effects of continued moisture mismanagement. The clinical differences between pressure ulcers and continence lesions are listed in Table14.1.

Prevention is better than cure

As always, prevention is better than cure. Therefore, to begin with, as far as possible, it is vital to address the cause of the incontinence (or sweating, or both). This may include instigating a regular toileting regime (e.g. 2–3 hourly) and excellence in skin care in the event that incontinence occurs. In any event it is essential that expert advice is sought from a Continence Specialist Nurse who will be able to assess, treat and manage the cause of the incontinence. In the meantime, the following care must be provided to avoid moisture lesions:

1 instigate a 2–3 hourly toileting regime
2 instigate a repositioning regime (a and b can be achieved together)
3 use of appropriate size and type of continence pad; these must be fitted to the conformity of the body and should not be placed as a sheet under the patient
4 good standards of personal hygiene; keeping the patient clean and dry
5 the use of an appropriate moisture barrier creams/sprays that will assist in preventing moisture sitting next to the skin
6 ensure adequate nutrition and hydration.

15 Vascular disease

Figure 15.1   A healthy and a diseased artery

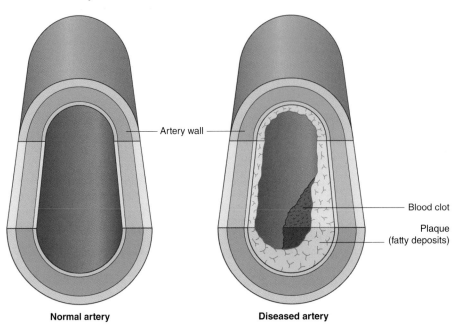

Normal artery   Diseased artery

Figure 15.2   Location of foot pulses

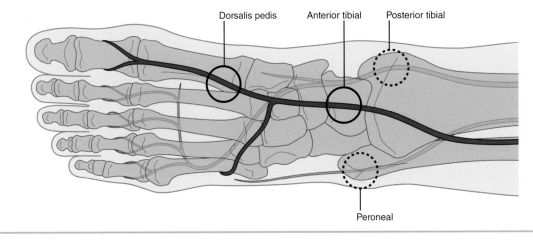

Wound Care at a Glance, First Edition. Ian Peate and Wyn Glencross. © 2015 John Wiley & Sons, Ltd. Published 2015 by John Wiley & Sons, Ltd.
Companion website: www.ataglanceseries.com/nursing/woundcare

Vascular disease, also known as arterial insufficiency, is the lack of adequate arterial blood supply to a certain organ(s) or part(s) of the body, which can result in reduced tissue viability or tissue death. The most common type of vascular disease seen in wound care is ulceration to the lower limbs due to vascular insufficiency, where limb pain and ulceration may occur due to this lack of blood supply; however, similar problems can develop in the upper limbs.

Lower limb ulcers (arterial ulcers) are the most common type of chronic wound, as many will either be very slow to heal or will not heal at all due to varying degrees of reduced or no blood supply to the limb, or parts of the limb.

Aetiology

Approximately 20% of all lower limb ulceration will be due to vascular disease, with the remainder due to venous disease or a combination of venous and arterial disease. Once a mixed aetiology exists it is the more serious arterial disease that must take priority in terms of treatment. Potential common causes of arterial insufficiency include diabetes mellitus (usually microvascular disease) and rheumatoid arthritis, and can affect any age group.

Arteriosclerosis is a term used for the thickening and hardening of the arterial walls caused by cholesterol deposits that build up on the inside wall of the artery/capillary, gradually narrowing the lumen through which blood travels, thereby reducing the blood supply to the surrounding tissues. It is considered most common in elderly people; other predisposing factors for arteriosclerosis are known to be obesity, hyperglycaemia, hypertension, hypercholesterolemia, smoking and a sedentary lifestyle. Figure 15.1 shows a healthy and a diseased artery.

Buerger's disease (i.e. thromboangiitis), which is strongly associated with smoking tobacco, is a condition that develops through recurring inflammation, clotting and vaso-occlusion (narrowing of the medium or large arteries and veins due to the inflammation) caused by the carbon in tobacco, thereby leading to a reduced circulation. This condition commonly affects smokers between the ages of 20 and 40 years, and is thought to cause an immune response to tobacco in those who are susceptible.

Additional factors that must be considered

Due consideration must be given to the possible presence of generalized vascular disease in patients who have had a cerebra-vascular accident (stroke) (by the development of a clot in the brain), those with vascular dementia, cardiovascular disease (e.g. angina and coronary artery disease), those who are given certain drugs, such as inotropes, that are commonly used in critically ill patients, and those with vascular diseases of vital organs such as the kidneys. Although in these conditions arterial insufficiency is usually restricted to the specific arteries, there is a possibility that the condition may be widespread affecting other arteries and capillaries. If for example a major artery is occluded due to hypertension (resulting in a stroke), it is possible that the smaller arteries and/or capillaries in the skin could be affected, making the patient more vulnerable to pressure damage or delayed healing of other wound types.

Nursing staff must therefore be extra vigilant in maintaining skin integrity in any patient with any of the aforementioned conditions as the likelihood of them developing wounds anywhere on the body with resulting poor healing rates is too great a risk to ignore. In such cases where a wound does occur it is vital that the patient is referred for an accurate diagnosis so that causes of delayed healing can be identified and addressed if possible.

Diagnostic tests for arterial disease

The following are common tests for measuring arterial insufficiency of the extremities:

Pulses – peripheral pulses must be assessed for all extremity wounds. However as a decreased blood supply may be affecting the limb (causing a wound) it is possible that the pulse may not be palpated. When checking a pulse by palpation, the rhythm, regularity and strength must be noted. The pulses to be palpated are the femoral, popliteal, dorsalis pedis and posterior tibial pulse of the leg; the brachial and radial pulses of the arm must be palpated in the case of arm ulceration. If pulses are not palpable, they may be heard via Doppler ultrasound. Figure 15.2 shows the location of main foot pulses.

Doppler ultrasound – this involves listening to the sound of the blood pulsating through the arteries using a hand-held device. The sound indicates the patency of the artery. A healthy artery has 2 or 3 beats that occur as the artery expands and contracts with the flow of blood. These are known as triphasic and biphasic beats. If the artery is compromised it will usually have only one beat (monophasic) that sounds loud and is 'gushing' or a 'wind tunnel' sound. This identifies a narrowing, occlusion or hardening (calcification) of the artery.

Ankle–brachial pressure index (ABPI) – This involves non-invasive assessment of the blood pressures in all four limbs and each of three arteries of the feet. A calculation is carried out that provides the ratio of the systolic blood pressure of the lower extremities compared to the upper extremities. This establishes an ABPI measurement that indicates the amount of blood that is travelling through each artery, or not, as the case may be. This is discussed in greater detail in a later chapter.

Capillary refill – this is a simple test that is a reliable indicator of surface arterial blood flow (i.e. to the skin, tips of digits) and involves pressing on the distal tip of the toe (or finger) for 5 seconds (i.e. emptying surface blood vessels). Capillary refill time is recorded based on the time it takes to refill and regain its original colour. A normal refill time is 3 seconds. A delayed refill time could indicate arterial insufficiency.

Rubor of dependency (Buerger's test) – briefly, this is a non-invasive test that involves lying the patient supine and noting the colour of the plantar aspect of the foot (the sole). The limb is elevated at varying degrees up and the colour of the plantar foot is noted. A healthy circulation will not change in colour even at a 60° elevation.

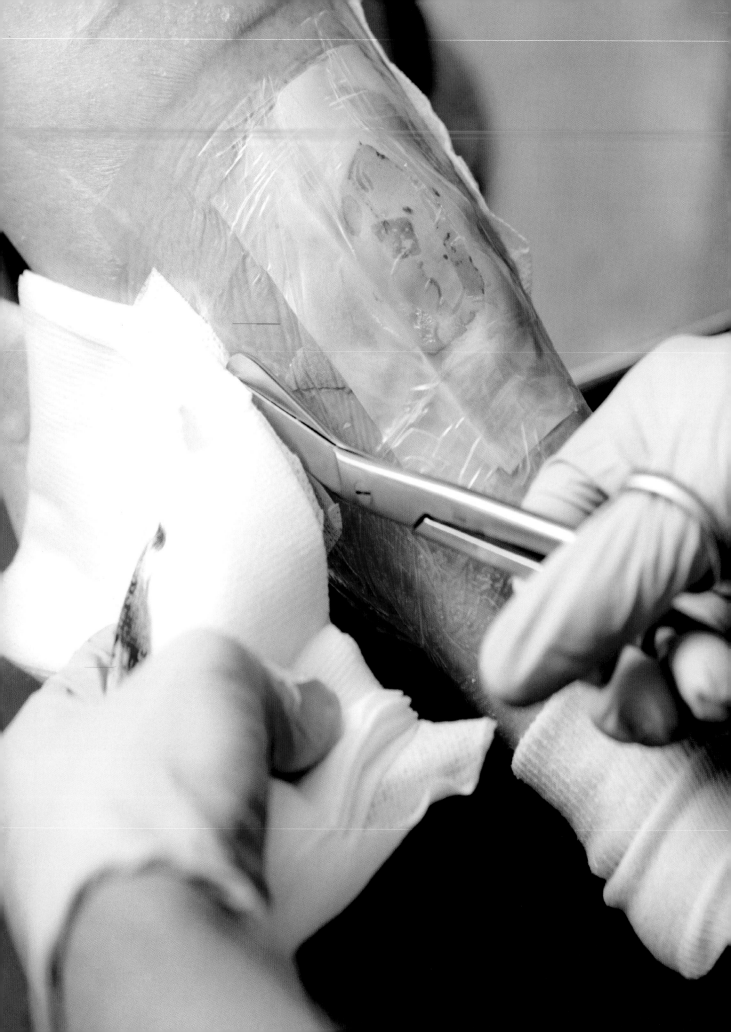

Wound management in practice

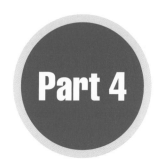

Part 4

Chapters

Visit the companion website at www.ataglanceseries.com/nursing/woundcare to test yourself on these topics.

Assessment of skin

Figure 16.1 The history

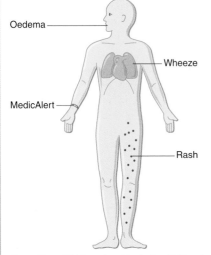

What's the trouble ?????

I'm telling you the diagnosis

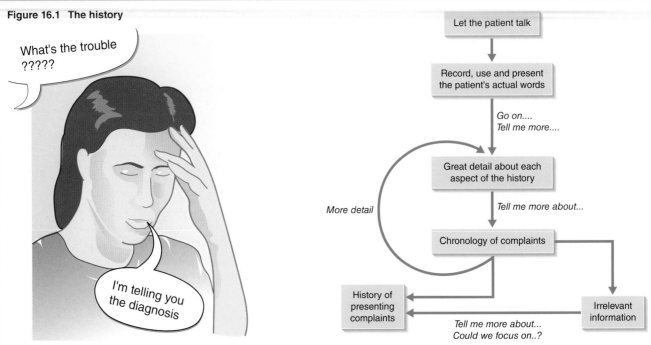

Let the patient talk

Record, use and present the patient's actual words

Go on....
Tell me more....

Great detail about each aspect of the history

More detail

Tell me more about...

Chronology of complaints

History of presenting complaints

Tell me more about...
Could we focus on..?

Irrelevant information

Source: Davey 2014, figure from Chapter 5, p. 10. Reproduced with permission of Wiley & Sons, Ltd.

Figure 16.2 The assessment

Oedema

Wheeze

MedicAlert

Rash

- Scalp and hair

- Face (include eyes, nose and mouth)

- Ears and neck (the outer ear, external ear. Examine the neck and feel for any enlarged lymph nodes)

- Chest and abdomen (examine breasts and axillae and feel for any enlarged lymph nodes)

- Back and buttocks

- Arms, hands and fingernails (inspect web spaces, distinguished lesions on the dorsum of the hand and the palms; look at the cuticles and the periungual area)

- Legs, feet and toenails (examine the feet the same way you will have examined the hands)

- Genitalia (feel for any enlarged lymph nodes in the groin)

Source: Davey 2014, figure from Chapter 6, p. 12. Reproduced with permission of Wiley & Sons, Ltd.

Wound Care at a Glance, First Edition. Ian Peate and Wyn Glencross. © 2015 John Wiley & Sons, Ltd. Published 2015 by John Wiley & Sons, Ltd.
Companion website: www.ataglanceseries.com/nursing/woundcare

The skin is the largest organ of the body and one of the most important. Throughout the lifespan a person's skin is subjected to a large number of insults; these can be both internal and external and can affect either its structure or function. In a healthy person the skin is strong, resilient and has the ability to repair itself in response to all but the most severe of insults. However, skin may be subject to changes that result in it becoming vulnerable, impaired and dysfunctional. Some of the changes are intrinsic, for example the effects of skin conditions, ageing or underlying illness, and others are extrinsic and include environmental damage.

Patient history

One of the most important aspects of assessing the skin is to ensure that a detailed history is taken eliciting the most salient and important aspects of the patient's story. The amount of time required to take a meaningful history will depend upon the person's complaint. Taking the history should receive the most time during the consultation and the time allocated to undertake this essential aspect of the discussion should reflect this. A comprehensive assessment is required.

Diagnosing the underlying cause of a wound is essential. The cause of the wound must be identified; if it is a chronic wound then the underlying factors that may have contributed to or are contributing to the chronicity should be identified so that they can be controlled.

The history provides you with an essential insight into the key features of the complaint and this must be recorded and where the patient provides information this should be recorded in her or his own words not masked by medical jargon. The most important skill is to listen and let or encourage the patient to talk, without interruption. Ask open questions so as to elicit as much information as possible, you may also be required to ask closed questions so as to get to the point or seek clarification. If the patient is not able to provide primary data then secondary sources of data will be required; for example, ask relatives, other healthcare professionals or consult the person's health records (Figure 16.1).

The history and summary of your findings must be recorded in the patient's notes. It is also useful to provide the patient with a summary of your findings to ensure that you have got it right.

Past medical history

This is a crucial aspect of the history and should be recorded in detail in chronological order

Drug history

Determine what medications the patient is taking and ask them why they are taking them, even if you know what the drug is usually prescribed for. Are these medications prescribed or are they over the counter or herbal remedies? If the person is using topical medications ascertain what these are and why they are using them and how they are using them.

Allergies

Establish if the patient has any allergies; you should ask them if they are allergic to anything. Obtain a detailed description of the allergic response to medication or any allergens, for example specific dressings, latex gloves. Find out the precise nature of the allergy. Any allergies must be clearly recorded in the person's notes and on drug charts, some people wear medicalert type identifiers, for example bracelets or pendants.

Smoking

The association between cigarette smoking and delayed wound healing is well recognized in clinical practice. Ask the patient if they smoke or have ever smoked, what type how many and for how long. In a respectful manner you can remind the person about the risks of smoking; this may help them give up.

Alcohol use

Alcohol consumption can increase the risk of infection and interfere with wound closure. Estimating alcohol consumption can help determine if intake is a potential risk factor.

Physical assessment of the skin

Examination of the skin must go hand in hand with the taking of a detailed history (Figure 16.2).

Ensure a good light source is available when examining the skin; the patient should be positioned in such a way that you can examine them and they are comfortable; only expose the relevant areas. There are a number of reasons why an assessment or examination of the skin is needed. A number of disease states can be shown on the skin. Findings can represent a disease process that is limited exclusively to the skin or there may be evidence of systematic disease. Skin lesions are numerous and present in infinite variations, careful examination and a detailed history will help to determine if the findings are skin only or systemic in nature.

You may be required to:

- inspect
- palpate
- percuss
- auscultate.

Examination should include all body surfaces and examination of the skin, nails and hair should take place as well as the mucous membranes. An entire body examination is not needed if there is a readily recognised lesion (a localized process); however, findings may be missed if you do not look beyond the most apparent pathology or if you do not listen to what it is that is troubling the person. A systematic approach to skin assessment should be adopted and a head to toe approach is recommended. A body map should be used to document findings.

Assessment tools

There are a variety of tools that can be used to undertake an assessment of the skin. Common tools in use are predictors of risk, risk assessment tools and are related to the assessment and prevention of pressure ulcers. A combination of intrinsic and extrinsic factors can result in the formation of a pressure ulcer. Definitions of pressure ulcers and guidelines concerning assessment and treatment have been provided by the National Pressure Ulcer Advisory Panel and the European Pressure Ulcer Advisory Panel.

The Waterlow pressure ulcer risk assessment/prevention policy tool is the most commonly used assessment tool in the UK, it is also the most easily understood. The tool is intended for use by a number of healthcare professionals and carers. When using Waterlow or any other risk assessment tool the practitioner must also exercise their professional judgement in determining the risk status of the patient.

17 # Assessment of the patient with a wound

Figure 17.1 The inverted pyramid approach to wound assessment

It is the whole of the patient that needs to be assessed when managing wounds, not simply the 'hole' in the patient - using the following order:

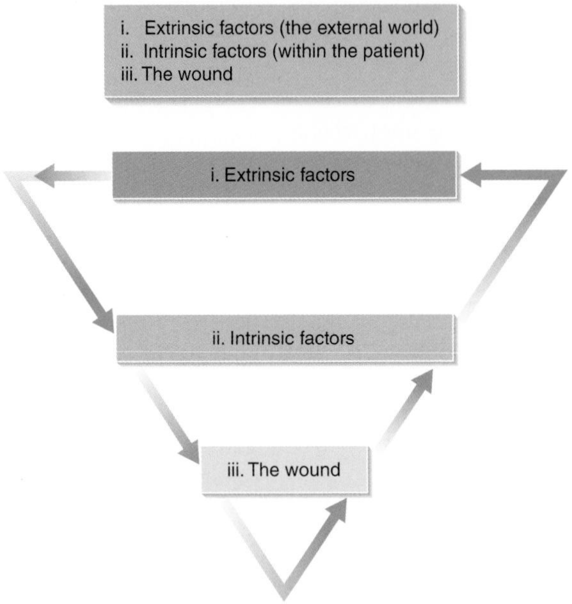

> i.   Extrinsic factors (the external world)
> ii. Intrinsic factors (within the patient)
> iii. The wound

i. Extrinsic factors

ii. Intrinsic factors

iii. The wound

Figure 17.2 The Nursing Process

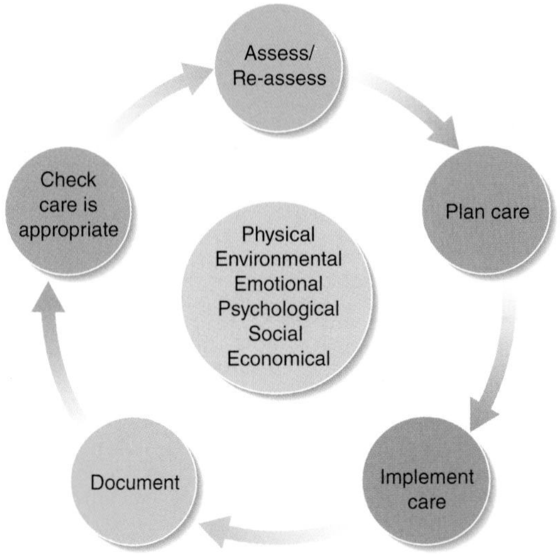

Assess/
Re-assess

Plan care

Check
care is
appropriate

Physical
Environmental
Emotional
Psychological
Social
Economical

Document

Implement
care

Wound Care at a Glance, First Edition. Ian Peate and Wyn Glencross. © 2015 John Wiley & Sons, Ltd. Published 2015 by John Wiley & Sons, Ltd.
Companion website: www.ataglanceseries.com/nursing/woundcare

Many nurses make the common mistake of looking at and noting the condition of the wound without first considering the patient as a whole, or at all. They apply dressing/treatments to a wound that may be contra-indicated for a medical condition he/she may have as they have failed to consider the patient holistically. For example, they may regularly change the dressing type because the wound is not progressing as it should, which could be that the patient is not eating sufficient amounts to promote healing. The nurse thinks that the wound will eventually heal if she selects the 'right' dressing and so continually tries different products on the wound without achieving her desired aim. This nurse has failed to consider the patient holistically and as a result of that failure the wound does not progress as it should.

A doctor would not prescribe a treatment/drug without first considering the patient holistically, as the failure to do so could cause potential harm or a reaction due to contra-indications, and the same principle applies to wound management.

This chapter will therefore consider the importance of assessing the patient holistically rather than simply assessing the wound only. It will consider the factors that affect healing already discussed in Chapters 10 and 11, and will promote a systematic approach to wound assessment to ensure the patient is considered as a whole rather than simply treating the 'hole' in the patient.

The inverted pyramid approach to wound assessment

This process is a 360° ongoing cycle of assessment that continually considers anything that could be delaying the wounds progression to healing. It is a process that when documented, provides evidence to the multidisciplinary team about the wounds progress and any factors that could be hindering that process (Figure 17.1).

1 *Extrinsic factors*

First stop and consider the environment the patient is being nursed in: who is providing nutrition, if anyone? What type of nutrition is that? What type of equipment is the patient being nursed on? Is he being turned regularly and is this recorded on a chart? What about his clothing or footwear: are they ill fitting? Is the patient still smoking to excess? Is the patient or a relative interfering with the dressings being applied?

Many extrinsic factors that are preventing a wound from healing can be improved upon once it has been identified and given due consideration as part of this process. For example the patient with the pressure ulcer whose wound is not improving because inadequate pressure relieve is not being provided will have improved healing rates once frequent position changes are introduced; in other words, the cause of the wound has been identified on assessment and adequately addressed (as far as possible) in order to improve healing rates.

2 *Intrinsic factors*

Next it is important that you consider any underlying medical conditions the patient may have and as far as you can deal with these; for example, the patient may be a diabetic and it is crucial that blood sugar levels are monitored and maintained within acceptable levels (i.e. around 5mmls) in order to encourage wound healing. Many medical conditions are out of your control; however, it is vital as far as is possible to manage these appropriately.

Many intrinsic factors are unchangeable, such as age for example. However others can be improved upon such as quality of nutrition. However, it must be remembered that some medical conditions will mean that they can't be addressed and therefore the wound will not heal; for example, in cases of inoperable peripheral vascular disease, when the circulation is so limited that the limb is dying due to ischaemia. In such cases it is vital that the wound environment is maintained to its optimum condition-based on the aforementioned assessments.

3 *Wound assessment*

Once the above two steps in the process have been completed it is then essential to assess the wound itself; this will include noting the anatomical site of the wound, the dimensions and depth of the wound, the tissue type on the wound (e.g. granulation tissues, slough, necrosis); condition of the surrounding skin; levels and type of exudate oozing from the wound; signs of maceration or excoriation; signs of infection and pain levels, including aggravating factors for pain.

The above findings must then be recorded on wound chart that lists each of the above (see Figure 20.1). Reassessments of the wound, along with the extrinsic and intrinsic assessments ought to be carried out at intervals determined appropriate for that wound type, healing rate and health care setting the patient is nursed in.

Frequency of assessment

It is a minimum expectation that a wound is reassessed (using the above process) weekly in the hospital or nursing home setting, and monthly as a minimum in the community setting (e.g. by district nurses) (Figure 17.2). The frequency however must be determined by the nurses who are responsible for the patients wound management. If the wound is slow to heal due to age and poor circulation for example, then fortnightly or monthly reassessments will be necessary providing all factors influencing the healing rate has been recognised and addressed. Until such time then weekly assessments are essential. When a wound is infected more frequency assessments will be necessary in order to monitor for potential systemic infection that would render the patient very unwell, and would require medical intervention.

18 Classification of wounds

Figure 18.1   An acute wound (laceration)

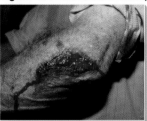

Figure 18.2   A chronic wound (leg ulcer)

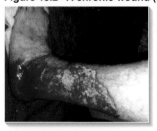

Figure 18.3   A necrotic wound (black)

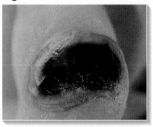

Figure 18.4   A sloughy wound (yellow)

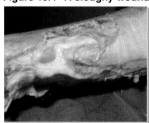

Figure 18.5   An infected wound (green)

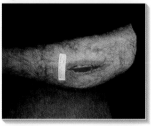

Figure 18.6   A granulating wound (red)

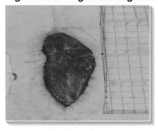

Figure 18.7   An epithelializing wound (pink)

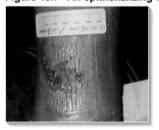

Wound Care at a Glance, First Edition. Ian Peate and Wyn Glencross. © 2015 John Wiley & Sons, Ltd. Published 2015 by John Wiley & Sons, Ltd.
Companion website: www.ataglanceseries.com/nursing/woundcare

The classification of wounds can be placed into two main categories; acute and chronic. There are two subcategories that identify the phases of the wound healing process and the tissue type(s) on the wound bed at any given time. The classification of wounds enables nursing staff to accurately assess and plan care for any given wound taking into consideration the holistic assessment of the patient. It therefore may become evident on assessment of the patient that an acute wound will undoubtedly become chronic due to underlying co-morbidities in some cases. There is no definite way to classify wounds; however, the inclusion of the following on a wound assessment form will enable nursing staff to utilize a tool that is neither too simplistic nor complex in order to identify key aspects relating to any given wound so that appropriate care can be planned.

Acute wounds

An acute wound is induced by trauma or surgery. There are many different causes of trauma, as listed below:

Incision – sometimes described as a 'cut'; this wound is usually induced by a sharp object (e.g. scalpel, knife, shard of glass or a metal sheet) that causes a 'slice' to the skin. There is usually very little tissue loss and the edges are therefore usually very clearly defined. The depth can vary from superficial to deep.

Laceration/skin tear (Figure 18.1) – this is usually caused by a blow against a blunt object that causes the skin to 'split'. Often there is swelling and some tissue loss. It often creates a skin flap that can be very thick or very thin in depth. A *skin tear* is usually caused by the tearing of the skin by a sharp object such as a nail, a fingernail, or by clothing/belts or rough handling. The frail elderly skin is often subject to this type of trauma. The depth is usually superficial and confined to the skin, but can affect deeper tissues.

Burn – can be caused by heat (fire), cold (frostbite), chemicals (Figure 18.3) and electricity. It is vital to identify the cause of the burn in order to treat it appropriately. It can vary in depth from superficial to deep.

Scald – can be caused by hot liquids and steam and must be quickly cooled. The damage can vary in depth from superficial to deep.

Puncture – a penetrating wound that can be of varying depth caused by pointed objects such as nails, wooden stakes, pins, needles, teeth (e.g. cat bites). These can appear insignificant due to the small opening on the skin, but underlying structural damage and infection are risk with this wound type. It is possible that a puncture of the skin can occur when a broken bone penetrates the skin.

Contusion – is a bruise caused by rupture of superficial blood vessels caused by the trauma, with no break to the skin itself. The bruising will disperse in around 14 days via the venous and lymphatic drainage so requires no topical treatments. The darker the discolouration is, the deeper the damage usually.

Friction – is the erosion of superficial (and sometimes deeper) tissues caused by the sudden or constant rubbing of the skin against a rougher surface. This type of wound requires healing by secondary intention.

Pressure – this is tissue death that creates a wound, which is caused by unrelieved and prolonged pressure applied against the skin.

Shearing – this is a closed wound where tissues attached to bone are torn away from the bone due to opposing forces of two tissue types. The affects are deep seated and can be painful due to inflammation of the bursa tissues at the site of trauma (bursitis). This type of injury is not usually visible to the eye, but will make the patient more vulnerable to rapid onset of pressure damage.

Chronic wounds

A chronic wound is defined as a being induced by a variety of causes and does not progress through the phases of wound healing leading to a prolonged or static wound due to underlying causes, usually of a duration longer than 6 weeks. The following wound types may become chronic, but any wound from any cause can become chronic due to underlying factors that affect the healing rates:

- leg ulcers (venous or arterial ulceration) (Figure 18.2)
- diabetic foot ulceration
- pressure ulcer
- some skin conditions (e.g. eczema, psoriasis, blistering).

Tissue types

The aim of wound management is to prevent the build-up of unwanted tissues types on the wound bed, while encouraging the growth of granulation and epithelial (healing) tissue in order to repair the wound. Tissue types are commonly documented in the following colours that can be used as part of documentation, which will be expanded on in future chapters. The types of tissue commonly found on a wound bed are:

Necrotic tissue (Figure 18.3) – (black) wet or dry tissue adhered to the wound bed consisting of red blood cells, skin cells, bacteria, varying levels of wound exudate (if moist or wet), and any other debris that may be on the wound such as dressing fibres or foreign bodies. Necrotic tissue can also consist of gangrene (tissue death) and it is important for the nurse to identify what type of necrotic tissue is on the wound, and this will also be discussed later. This is unwanted tissue.

Slough (Figures 18.4 and 18.5) – (yellow) wet or dry tissue consisting of congealed wound exudate, debris, skin cells, bacteria and blood cells. The actual colour of slough will vary depending on the ingredients within it. For example a grey slough will have red blood cells, while a yellow slough (Figure 18.4) will have many white blood cells within it. A green slough (Figure 18.5) will have a bacterium known as pseudomonas within it; however, it must be pointed out that infection is not identified by the colour of slough (discussed later). This is unwanted tissue.

Granulation tissue (Figure 18.6) – (red) this is wanted tissue, and consists of angiogenesis (new blood vessels) utilized in tissue repair. The aim is to maintain a 'red' granulating wound while preventing the build-up of unwanted tissue types.

Epithelial tissue (Figure 18.7) – (pink) this tissue type demonstrates the covering of skin over the granulation tissue as the wound fills with new tissues. Once the wound is entirely covered with epithelial tissue the wound is regarded as closed (healed).

19 Legal and ethical aspects of wound care

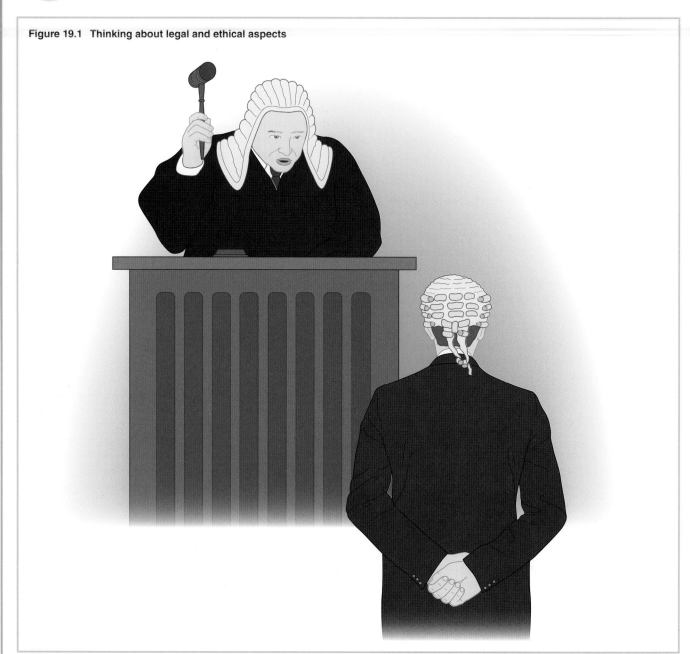

Figure 19.1 Thinking about legal and ethical aspects

All registered nurses are accountable to the Nursing and Midwifery Council (NMC), to their employer and to the law. All untrained nursing staffs are accountable to their employer and to the law. If the untrained nurse works under the supervision of a registered nurse the registered nurse will also be accountable for the untrained nurses' actions. However, all staff are accountable to the patient at any time, and this therefore means that nursing staff must endeavour to adhere to legislation and professional codes of conduct, and must at all times act in the 'best interests' of the patient. With this thought, let us now consider how these professional and legal expectations affect the wound care that we provide to our patients.

Professional standards

According to the NMC, good record keeping and care planning is a 'non-negotiable skill that all registered nurses must possess'. They consider it equally as important as any other clinical skill required to fulfil the role of a registered nurse. It is commonly regarded that poor standards in documentation is a reflection on the standards of care provided, which would therefore be regarded as equally as bad as the standards evidenced in the records.

In May 2008 the NMC released the revised code of conduct that all registered nurses and midwifes must adhere to: 'The Code: Standard of conduct, performance and ethics for nurses and midwives'. This Code states 'People in your care must be able to trust you with their health and wellbeing. To justify that trust, you must:

• Make the care of people your first concern, treating them as individuals and respecting their dignity
• Work with others to protect and promote the health and wellbeing of those in your care, their families and carers, and the wider community
• Provide a high standard of practice and care at all times
• Be open and honest, act with integrity and uphold the reputation of your profession.'
The Code continues to state:
• As a professional, you are personally accountable for actions and omissions in your practice and must always be able to justify your decisions
• You must always act lawfully, whether those laws relate to your professional practice or personal life
• Failure to comply with this Code may bring your fitness to practice into question and endanger your registration
• This Code should be considered together with the NMC's rules, standards guidance and advice available.

In brief, this means that nursing staff when dealing with wounds, must first obtain valid consent before treating a patient; they must respect confidentiality, delegate effectively, use the best evidence available, keep their skills and knowledge up to date, act with integrity, keep clear and accurate records and utilize the expertise of others when it is appropriate. Those records will assist with continuity of care and will be utilised by all members of the multi-disciplinary team. The failure to adhere to these standards could lead to professional sanctions against the nurse, including a 'Striking Off [the register] Order'. It is therefore an expectation that all registered general nurses will be competent in the management of non-complex wounds at the point of entry on the NMC Register.

Legal standards

It is vital that registered nurses ensure that contemporaneous records are kept and that the NMC standards on record keeping are adhered to at all times. Where documentation is required from untrained staff, it is wise that they too follow the aforementioned principles. At any point in time those documents could be seized by the police or by the Coroner; they may be requested by the patient and/or the patient's family for use in litigation and therefore the Courts, or by the CQC during an inspection of the care setting, all of whom will scrutinise the evidence within those documents.

You may be required to account for your practice, often several years later, and you will need to rely on your documentation to do this, so it is not only in the patient's interests but in your own to ensure you maintain high standards of documentation at all times in accordance with the standards expected. This means that nursing staff are required to produce documentary evidence of the care they have provided to every patient they are responsible for. However, it is commonly stated by members of the nursing/care professions that 'if it isn't written down, then it did not happen', yet despite this common awareness, nursing documentation on the whole is generally poor.

Tissue viability issues commonly scrutinized

Complaints and litigation are on the increase in most care sectors. Common issues are regarding (but not limited to) the prevention and treatment of pressure ulcers; general wound care and wound infections that may have led to sepsis, unnecessary pain and suffering, or even death; suspected abuse or neglect, particularly of elderly people who present with skin tears, bruising and pressure ulcers; poor skin integrity due to poor nutrition and incontinence.

The standard of care provided will be judged by a Court based on the documentary evidence available and expert opinion. In reaching this judgement each nurse involved in the case will be measured against the responsible body of registered nurses skilled in tissue viability, who would not fail to adhere to the standards expected in tissue viability practice at the given time, and to the NMC Code of Conduct and Standards in Record Keeping.

If it is found by a Court that there was a failure in the duty of care by the nurse or carers (due to lack of documentary evidence to argue otherwise), it is most common that compensation is paid to the Claimant by vicarious liability (insurance policy). The employer may then use their own disciplinary procedures against the nurse, or they may refer the nurse to the NMC. In the most serious of cases sanctions could include imprisonment of the nurse/carer for Wilful Neglect, Assault and Battery or Abuse.

20 Documenting wounds and keeping records

	Initial assessment date	Evaluation date	Evaluation date	Evaluation date	Evaluation date	Evaluation date	Evaluation date
Wound Assessment Chart (Use a separate chart for every wound) Patient ID_____ Wound Type_____ Wound Site_____							
Wound presentation % N – Necrotic (black) G – Granulation (bright red) S – Sloughy (yellow) E – Epithelialisation (pink)							
Exudate colour 1 – Straw colour 2 – Blood-stained 3 – Purulent *							
Level of exudate 4 – None 5 – Minimal (contained within primary dressing) 6 – Moderate (extends to secondary dressing) 7 – High (secondary dressing saturated)							
Other clinical signs of infection 1 – Non-healing / deterioration 5 – Bleeding 2 – Increased exudate 6 – Malodour 3 – Increased pain 7 – Pus 4 – Increased erythema							
Wound Traced? Yes or No (please circle)	Y / N	Y / N	Y / N	Y / N	Y / N	Y / N	Y / N
Wound photographed? Yes or No (please circle)	Y / N	Y / N	Y / N	Y / N	Y / N	Y / N	Y / N
Consent for photography obtained? (please circle)	Y / N	Y / N	Y / N	Y / N	Y / N	Y / N	Y / N
Wound Dimensions – width, depth, length (cms) **EPUAP Grade of Pressure Ulcer** 1 – Increasing * 2 – Decreasing 3 – Static * (review treatment)							
Doppler Ultrasound assessment carried out? (for leg ulcers) Yes or No	Y / N	Y / N	Y / N	Y / N	Y / N	Y / N	Y / N
Wound odour (a) none (b) malodorous *							
Wound Infection - are there 2 or more clinical signs? Yes or No (circle)	Y / N	Y / N	Y / N	Y / N	Y / N	Y / N	Y / N
Wound swab taken? Yes or No (please circle)	Y / N	Y / N	Y / N	Y / N	Y / N	Y / N	Y / N
Antibiotics Prescribed? Yes or No (please circle) (refer to path report)	Y / N	Y / N	Y / N	Y / N	Y / N	Y / N	Y / N
Condition of wound margins e.g. flat, raised, irregular, undermined							
Condition of surrounding skin 1 – Healthy 4 – Oedematous * 7 – Dermatitis / Eczema 2 – Inflamed * 5 – Blistered 3 – Macerated 6 – Ischaemic							
Pain assessment score (see pain assessment documentation)							
Onset of pain caused by? (e.g. walking, dressing change. Please state)							
Pain is relieved by? (e.g. analgesia, elevation. Please state)							
Signature & Designation							

Patient's own description of the pain: ....

....

....

....

Additional Information: ....

....

....

Wound Care at a Glance, First Edition. Ian Peate and Wyn Glencross. © 2015 John Wiley & Sons, Ltd. Published 2015 by John Wiley & Sons, Ltd.
Companion website: www.ataglanceseries.com/nursing/woundcare

In the previous chapter we have considered the professional and legal reasons why high documentation standards must be practised at all times and the implications if we fail to adhere to these standards. As we have already stated, good documentation is a non-negotiable skill that all nurses must possess according to the NMC, and yet there is an increase in successful litigants who won their case purely because the provision of care was not evidenced in the nursing records. Indeed this is a common occurrence seen in the most recent project by the Department of Health, known as 'Zero Tolerance of Avoidable Pressure Ulcers' and in cases of litigation on pressure ulcers (both discussed in later chapters).

It is therefore important to be clear on the rationale and variety of evidence we can produce in tissue viability in order to demonstrate the standard of care provided at any given time. But first we must refresh on the processes involved in producing this documentation.

The Nursing Process

In the 1970s Nancy Roper developed the concept of the Nursing Process using a nursing model that considered the patient holistically by assessing activities of daily living (ADLs) such as eating and drinking, breathing, eliminating and communication. She suggested that when assessing the patient the nurse must consider social, environmental, physical, economical, spiritual and psychological factors during the process. She argued that if this was done then no problem, need or risk would go unnoticed by the nurse, who would then be in a position to plan individualized, person-centred care for every health and social care need, problem or risk. The planned care would also include a realistic aim/goal, and instruction on how that care would be provided. The care must then be implemented and methods of implementation ought to be evidenced in the patient's documentation. The plan would set a review date where a reassessment of that specific problem, need or risk would be carried out in order to ensure appropriate care continues to be provided. Roper stated that if all ADLs are repeated at set dates (e.g. weekly/monthly) to create a continuous 360° cycle of Assessment, Planning, Implement, Evaluate (APIE), the patient would be confident that the necessary and appropriate care and/or intervention would be provided throughout their entire episode of care in any given care setting.

Tissue viability documentation

Following the Roper Principles, let us now consider how we can produce good standards in tissue viability documentation that would provide evidence of acceptable standards of care in accordance with a responsible body of registered nurse.

1 Assessment

Assessing a wound involves taking note of the wound's anatomical site; dimensions; depth (if a pressure ulcer, this will be by grade); tissue type on the wound; levels and type of wound exudate; condition of the surrounding skin (observing for maceration, excoriation, heat on touch and erythema, blistering or any other lesions), pain levels and aggravating or relieving factors of pain; and whether or not there is a malodour from the wound. This information can be recorded on a wound assessment chart (see Figure 20.1), by photography or by tracing the wound on acetate. All this documentation will provide monitoring that informs all members of the MDT.

2 Care planning

Once the assessment (or reassessment) is completed, the nurse can establish what the aims are to be in order to promote healing. A care plan can then be devised for each wound identified that instructs others on the management of each wound. The plan must include as a minimum identification of the site of the wound; the aim of the care plan; the type of dressing(s) to be applied to the wound; the frequency of dressing changes and a date when the wound must be reassessed. The plan must be clear and concise and should allow others to deliver the care that has been planned.

3 Implementing care

Wound care must be carried out using an aseptic technique, utilising sterile dressings. Once the care has been delivered this must be documented on the Evaluation chart, the content of which should reflect the directions on the care plan.

4 Check the care plan is appropriate

The dressing must be observed at least once on every shift for signs of wound exudate strike-through (i.e. the staining on the outer dressing). Whether or not there is any strike-through must then be recorded on the care plan evaluation document. Once the dressing shows evidence of strike-through, the dressing will require changing in order to avoid saturation and increased risk of a wound infection. On removal of the dressing the nurse must check the wound in order to establish whether or not the wound shows clinical changes and that the care plan remains appropriate if the findings are unchanged.

5 Making adaptations to the care plan

This may include increasing the frequency of dressing changes, or a different dressing choice to manage the exudate levels more appropriately. Rationale for any adaptations to the care plan must be documented in the care plan evaluation.

6 Reassessment

In the event the clinical findings are noted to have changed when re-dressing the wound (as detailed in Section 4 above) (e.g. increased exudate levels, signs of infection, increased pain, deterioration in the wound), the nurse must re-assess the wound once again (as stated in Section 1), and all findings must be recorded on the evaluation, and the care plan either amended or rewritten accordingly in order to reflect the changing requirements and aims of the wound.

In the event that no clinical changes are noted on daily checks or on dressing changes, then reassessment must be completed at intervals established by either clinical judgement or by weekly/fortnightly/monthly timeframes as stated by the 2010 Regulated Activities.

21 Evidence-based practice

Figure 21.1 Five stages associated with evidence-based practice

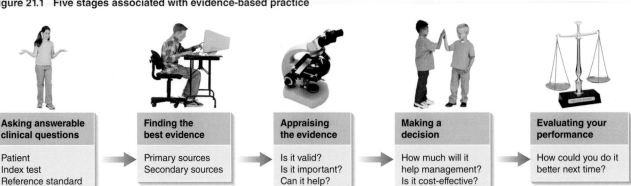

Asking answerable clinical questions	Finding the best evidence	Appraising the evidence	Making a decision	Evaluating your performance
Patient Index test Reference standard Target disorder	Primary sources Secondary sources	Is it valid? Is it important? Can it help?	How much will it help management? Is it cost-effective?	How could you do it better next time?

Source: Thompson and Van den Bruel 2011, figure on p. x of Introduction. Reproduced with permission of Wiley & Sons, Ltd.

Table 21.1 Hierarchy of evidence

Level	Description of evidence	Strength
I	Systematic review or meta-analysis of all relevant randomized controlled trials (RCTs), or evidence-based clinical practice guidelines based on systematic reviews of RCTs	Strongest
II	Evidence from at least one well-designed RCT	
III	Evidence from well-designed controlled trials without randomization	
IV	Evidence from well-designed case-control and cohort studies	
V	Systematic reviews of descriptive and qualitative studies	
VI	A single descriptive or qualitative study	
VII	The opinion of authorities and/or reports of expert committees	Weakest

Wound Care at a Glance, First Edition. Ian Peate and Wyn Glencross. © 2015 John Wiley & Sons, Ltd. Published 2015 by John Wiley & Sons, Ltd.
Companion website: www.ataglanceseries.com/nursing/woundcare

Because of the assortment of wound aetiologies along with their associated comorbidities, a variety of healthcare professionals from all health settings, with each one having a different knowledge base related to wound healing, deliver wound care. There is a need to standardize care and encourage optimal practice in wound management, with the key aim of improving patient outcomes. National guidelines for their management need to be developed. The background and justification for these guidelines provide the health professional with the rationale for their development associated with information relating to prevalence, potential patient outcomes and resource issues but they must be derived from an evidence base.

Practising evidence-based wound care will encourage practitioners to integrate valid and useful evidence with clinical expertise and each patient's unique features, enabling you to apply evidence to the treatment of patients.

Evidence-based wound care

Healthcare practice with a focus on wound care demands the highest level of evidence. Evidence-based wound management is the combination of best research evidence with clinical expertise and patient values. When a practitioner engages in evidence based practice they will be combining their expertise, acknowledging the patient's condition, using the best scientific evidence and listening to the patient's preference.

Wound care has often been taught through case examples and what was deemed best clinical practice. There are many elements of wound care that are, and in some instances continue to be, based on hearsay, custom and practice, with little thought being given to why things are done in a specific way.

With the increased importance of providing an evidence base to practice, there is now a need and a requirement to move away from indiscriminate clinical practice, experiential learning, associated with outmoded, unjustified opinions, to learning that has an evidence base. The evidence available extends from expert opinion to randomized clinical trials.

Healthcare practitioners (in line with clinical governance requirements) must strive to provide the safest and best quality care they can. Evidence based wound care practice requires thought along with a questioning approach to patient care. Evidence-based wound care is required because of the increasingly complex nature of health care and health care decisions, the requirement that services and treatments provided should be based on the best evidence of what works and what does not work and to be able to demonstrate adherence to codes of professional conduct.

Five stages of evidence-based practice

Evidence-based practice can be broken down into a number of stages. These are five stages associated with evidence-based practice (Figure 21.1).

The questions, asking answerable clinical questions

The first step is recognizing that there is a need for new information. This information need is likely to be vague and as such it will have to be converted into an answerable question in order to facilitate an efficient search for the answer. Precise answers can only be provided when a precise question has been posed. The question should be carefully framed, helping to determine what type

of evidence you will need to find. It is not unusual for a number of questions to emerge at the same time; it will not be possible to answer all of them at once. Failure to ask a focused and precise clinical question can be a major threat to evidence-based practice.

Acquiring the evidence, finding the evidence

Choosing the right evidence is of central importance. There are various sources of evidence, and it can be hard to know where to begin. The main sources of evidence often come from more experienced colleagues and textbooks, however there are problems with these sources of information. How can you be sure that the information colleagues provide is reliable? When using evidence from textbooks the opinions expressed may be out of date before the book is even published, or incompatible with current best evidence. A number of groups have established levels or hierarchies of evidence, usually based upon scientific merit in an empirical model. When examining the evidence it will be helpful to consider the hierarchy of evidence (Table 21.1).

Assessing the evidence, appraising

The evidence must be critically appraised to establish its validity and potential usefulness. The main questions to ask when appraising the evidence are:

- Can the evidence be trusted?
- What does the evidence mean?
- Does this answer the question?
- Is it relevant to practice?

There are different appraisal and interpreting skills that can be used depending on the kind of evidence being considered.

Arriving at a decision, acting on evidence

Once it has been decided that the evidence is of sound quality, another decision will need to be made whether the evidence should be incorporated into clinical practice – change. Consideration of both the benefits and risks of implementing the change, as well as the benefits and risks of excluding any alternatives should be undertaken. These decisions should be made in collaboration with the multidisciplinary team, managers and patients where appropriate. Resistance to change should be given serious consideration, as this can be a challenge. By involving all key stakeholders (colleagues, patients, carers, budget-holders, commissioners) can help ensure the change is implemented as well as sustained.

Evaluation and reflection, evaluation of performance

Evaluation and reflection are essential to determine whether the action(s) taken have achieved the desired results. This is a fundamental aspect of health care practice.

Evidence-based practice is a continuous, cyclical process. Once each stage of the process has been worked through it is likely that new questions will arise and will need to be answered. Evidence-based wound care should focus on employing a questioning approach to your practice. This should not be seen as a 'one-off' activity. It is a continuous process that can help you provide safe and high quality care to patients. An evidence-based approach can assist you in your own professional development as you question and seek evidence-based solutions.

22 Treatment options

Figure 22.1 Closure by primary intention

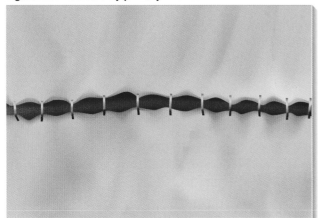

Source: P. Vong. Reproduced with permission of P. Vong

Figure 22.2 Closure by secondary intention

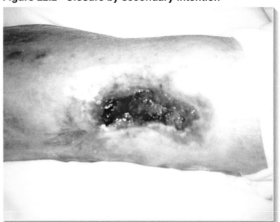

Figure 22.3 Larval therapy

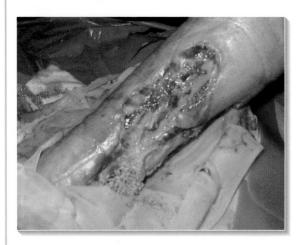

Figure 22.4 Topical negative pressure system, e.g. VAC negative pressure wound therapy

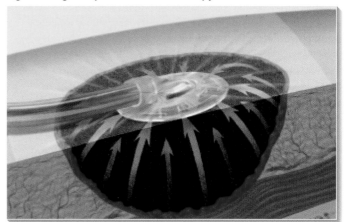

Source: KCI. Used with permission. Courtesy of KCI.

Wound closure

When a wound occurs, or when faced with a chronic wound, the assessing nurse must consider treatment options that will address the clinical findings of the wound and to promote healing rates. The choices made will depend on assessment of the wound as well as the patient. So, when a wound first occurs, the initial treatment option that must be considered is wound closure. There are two common types of closure.

Primary intention (Figure 22.1) – is the closure of a wound by the use of mechanical aids, such as sutures, staples, strips, glue or a combination of these to hold the edges of the wound together. It can only be used on wounds where there is little or no tissue loss where the margins of the wound can be held together by these aids without undue tension on them. If the tension on the aids is too great, the wound will dehisce (i.e. pull apart) and the wound will have a greater surface area requiring healing by the secondary intention.

Secondary (tertiary) intention – is when a wound is left 'open' and allowed to heal by contraction, without the use of mechanical aids other than dressings for a number of reasons; too much tissue loss to pull and hold the edges of the wound together; the wound has dehisced due to swelling, infection or too much tissue loss; primary intention is contraindicated due to a high risk of infection, particular common with abscesses and animal bites for example.

In either case the wound will progress through the phases of wound healing discussed in earlier chapters. The difference is that the healing can be visualised in wounds that heal by secondary intention, whereas with primary intention the healing rate occurs underneath the line of closure. In the meantime, a third method is used on occasions as follows.

Delayed primary intention – this is where a wound is initially allowed to heal by secondary intention and later closed by primary intention. The delay allows for reduction in swelling that could cause a wound to dehisce (e.g. a surgical wound), or it allows for treatment of infection in cases of abscesses or infected wounds (e.g. animal bites and boils that have been lanced). If an infected wound was closed by primary intention, for example, this would 'seal' in the bacteria that would multiply under the closure line, causing the wound to dehisce. Many experts argue that this type of closure should not be used in any event as once the wound surface area is colonized with bacteria, this will be sealed in when the wound is eventually closed. This type of closure must therefore be carefully considered.

Treatment options for secondary intention healing

If primary intention closure is not suitable, or if part of a wound closed by this method requires secondary intention closure, the next consideration for the nurse is to select the most appropriate treatment for the wound. The treatment options available will depend on the findings on wound and holistic patient assessment and on the aims of the wound at the given time. Let us now consider common options used in the UK.

Surgical debridement (Figure 22.2) – this is the mechanical removal of dead and devitalised tissue on the wound bed (e.g. necrosis, slough, gangrene) or the removal of infected tissues. It is carried out by a surgeon under an anaesthetic (local or a general) and may involve the removal of healthy tissue, so the wound may bleed. It is often carried out on wounds that require rapid cleansing due to infection or the risk of infection, particularly on the most vulnerable patients. However the risks of surgery must be weighed against the benefits of alternative methods, such as autolytic debridement.

Sharp debridement – is a method used by doctors, or nurses trained in this method to mechanically remove unwanted tissue from a wound (e.g. slough or necrosis). It can be done at the bedside and does not require an anaesthetic, and entails removal of dead tissue only. It does not involve cutting into healthy tissue so the wound should not bleed. Owing to this limitation it is not always possible to remove all of the unwanted tissue, and a combination of this and other methods may be required to fully debride the wound of unwanted tissue.

Larval therapy (Figure 22.3) – this is a method of tissue removal (slough, necrosis or gangrene) by the use of maggots. The larvae excrete an enzyme that liquefies the unwanted tissues. The larvae then drink this liquid thereby cleansing the wound bed. While drinking this liquid the larvae also swallow the bacteria present within the liquid, and the bacteria are then eradicated in the gut of the larvae. One treatment of larvae can remove a moderate amount of slough/necrosis; however, several treatments may be required before the wound is fully cleansed.

Autolytic debridement – this is a method of removal of dead and devitalized tissue on the wound bed (e.g. slough or necrosis) by the use of dressing products that create the optimum environment whereby the unwanted tissue is prevented in the first instance, or liquefied and absorbed into the dressing in the second, until the wound is fully cleansed of unwanted tissue types. In other words we are almost mimicking the action of maggots, but without using an enzyme. Instead we take advantage of the body's own moisture that exude onto the wound, and providing we maintain a moist environment on the wound, that moisture will liquefy unwanted tissue, whilst the dressing absorbs the excess liquid away. In cases where a wound is dry, or if the patient is dehydrated, we can use hydrating products to achieve the moist environment in order to kick-start the debridement process.

Topical negative pressure (Figure 22.4) – this is a method of wound healing that can only be used once the wound is free from dead and devitalised tissues, and usually follows any of the above methods of debridement. Negative pressure is applied to the wound bed, which then promotes an increase in the blood supply to the wound bed. This increases the rate of angiogenesis and therefore the growth of granulation tissue. It removes excess exudate, therefore maintaining a moist wound healing environment. As it removes the exudate it maintains minimal levels of bacteria on the wound bed, thereby reducing the risk of wound infection whilst it is in operation. Healing rates with this method are usually quicker than with traditional methods of healing. Topical negative pressure is also known as vacuum-assisted closure (VAC).

23 Pain management

Box 23.1 Comprehensive pain assessment summarized by the NOPQRST mnemonic

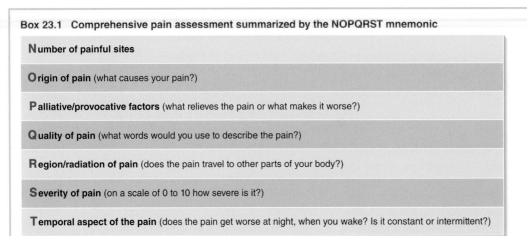

Number of painful sites

Origin of pain (what causes your pain?)

Palliative/provocative factors (what relieves the pain or what makes it worse?)

Quality of pain (what words would you use to describe the pain?)

Region/radiation of pain (does the pain travel to other parts of your body?)

Severity of pain (on a scale of 0 to 10 how severe is it?)

Temporal aspect of the pain (does the pain get worse at night, when you wake? Is it constant or intermittent?)

Figure 23.1 Visual analogue scales for pain assessment

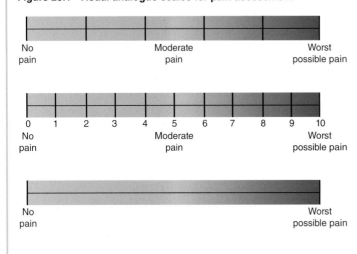

Figure 23.2 The WHO analgesic pain relief ladder, adapted from the World Health Organization

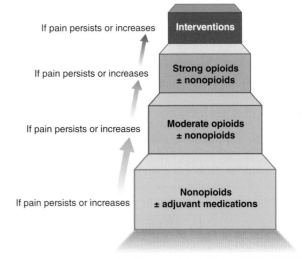

Pain – a holistic approach

Pain, just as it is with most issues in wound care can be complicated. Pain associated with a specific tissue injury that resolves in a time frame related to the degree of injury is acute pain. Chronic pain is less well defined and can be related to tissue damage (nociceptive pain) or nerve damage (neuropathic pain), or there may be a combination of the two. When infection is present this provides another pain dimension, and wound care interventions. The pain that patients experience can also be unrelated to the wound, for example rheumatoid pain, but related to wound care, specifically when positioning a patient for an intervention and the provision of analgesia. The pain experienced when a dressing is being changed is not therefore always limited to the wound itself. As well as the physical components of pain, there are also psychological and emotional factors exacerbating how a patient perceives pain. The various wound aetiologies bring with them different challenges related to pain and its consequences; for example, in diabetic neuropathy there is the absence of protective pain sensations, which can lead to significant tissue damage; the acute pain experienced by burns patients results in severe pain. Other challenges have to be faced in palliative wound care when this is related to advanced disease as the person nears the end of life. Pain management is a significant element of wound care, bringing with it a number of issues and challenges that require a sound evidence base and a multidisciplinary approach.

It is only in the last decade that there has been more appreciation of the role of pain in the life experience of those with wounds. Those patients with wounds such as leg ulceration are said to experience significantly greater bodily pain than the normal population, this phenomenon is not simply a consequence of an older population, it is more a feature of the wound in association with an underlying abnormal pain mechanism.

Wound-related pain

Wound-related pain can be described as an unpleasant symptom or unpleasant experience directly related to open skin, it can be background pain, i.e. chronic or persistent, that many be experienced most of the time. This is compared to an acute incident/procedure-related pain that can arise as a result of routine dressing changes or operative procedures such as biopsy or debridement. Pain is a subjective sensation that is best described by the patient as a result of their personal experience.

There are several individual factors that can influence the pain experience, including anxiety and pain expectation. Exacerbation of pain occurs when other local wound care factors are present including dressing change, wound cleansing, debridement, presence of infection, bacterial damage and inappropriate choice of dressing.

Unrelenting chronic background wound related pain can have a significant negative impact on the person's abilities to perform the activities of living, impacting on health and wellbeing . Experiencing wound related pain could be seen as one of the most devastating aspects of living with a chronic wound.

To minimize pain, various strategies (pharmacological and non-pharmacological) must be considered at the time of wound care related procedures including dressing change. A detailed assessment of pain is required so that plans may be put in place to anticipate pain-relieving needs, an evaluation on interventions must be carried out to determine effectiveness.

Pain assessment

It is an established fact that pain improves significantly with effective treatment, which promotes healing. Yet there are some instances where practitioners may be unconcerned or unwilling to accept the degree of suffering of patients from pain related to wounds. Assessing pain associated with wounds is a skill that must be underpinned by a sound knowledge base.

Wound-related pain can change over time, requiring frequent reassessment. Dressing change has been identified as the most painful aspect of wound care, as well as pain at rest between dressing changes and during the performance of daily activities. Pain assessment can help to distinguish the background pain from pain that is procedure provoked. Ongoing assessment of pain assessment can help to determine the temporal pain pattern for selecting and planning appropriate pain interventions, assess the efficacy of pain treatments/interventions, consider factors that may enhance or exacerbate wound-related pain and to identify barriers that can affect pain management.

Comprehensive pain assessment can be summarized by the mnemonic NOPQRST (Box 23.1). There is a selection of visual analogue scales available that will help the practitioner assess pain (Figure 23.1). It must be remembered that pain is not a one-dimensional experience; there are multiple factors that impact on pain and other important information is needed to ensure a holistic and thorough assessment has taken place. Providing patients with a list of words can help them describe the pain they are experiencing.

Pain management

Choosing the right treatment will depend on the outcome of the assessment. The practitioner should consider local treatment for pain as this brings with it less side effects. There are strategies that include the use of wound products that are moist, analgesia impregnated dressings and the application of topical analgesia.

There may also be a need to consider systemic treatment, this choice should not be solely based on size or type of wound; it must be based on the outcome of the assessment and need. Adherence to pain management protocols will guide treatment and the World Health Organization pain relief ladder provides a framework to work from, (Figure 23.2). Adjunct therapies such as muscle relaxants and steroids can be used to enhance effectiveness of analgesia. In some specific types of pain, such as neuropathic pain, anticonvulsants or tricyclic antidepressants can be used.

Emotional needs of the patient must be given consideration as pain associated with the wound coupled with the presence of a wound can trigger psychological distress. Psychological distress can cause explicit manifestations of stress, stress impacts on the ability of the body to heal; referral to a psychotherapist may be needed.

A key component of pain management associated with wounds is improving access to appropriate products, developing the knowledge base and undertaking a detailed holistic assessment of pain.

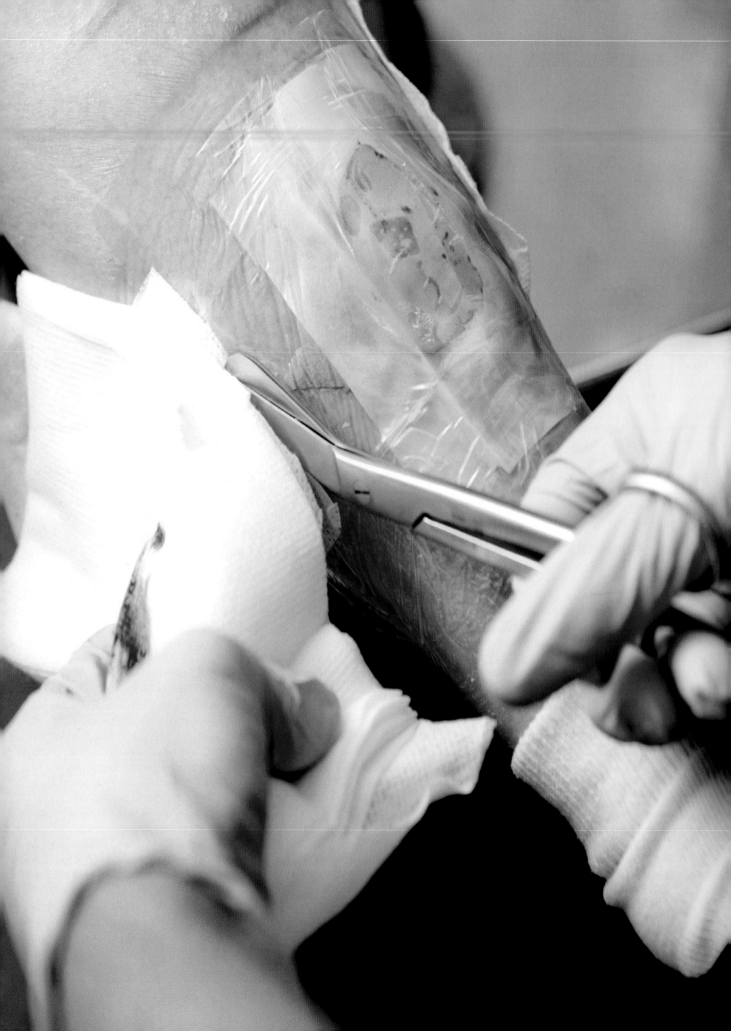

Dressing selection

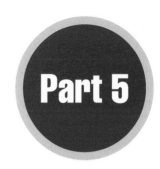

Part 5

 Visit the companion website at www.ataglanceseries.com/nursing/woundcare to test yourself on these topics.

(24) Principles of wound management I

Applying principles

Before a dressing or a treatment can be applied to a wound it is crucial that a full assessment is carried out (i.e. holistic and wound assessments). Any underlying causes of the wound must be addressed as far as possible and any factors that affect wound-healing rates must be dealt with as far as possible. This must be maintained on an ongoing basis. One classic error that tissue viability nurses frequently remark on is that nursing staff continually change the dressing or treatment believing that this will encourage the wound to heal, but fail to address the underlying cause or factors that hinder healing; for example with a pressure ulcer, nursing staff frequently fail to provide adequate pressure relief and/or fail to ensure a patient is eating sufficient nutrients that will promote healing, and then change the dressing type when the wound fails to heal. It must therefore be clear that it is the patient's own body that will heal the wound and not the dressing, which will simply provide an environment that will either promote healing rates if used appropriately or if not, the wound healing rates will be delayed.

The following principles must then be applied to the management of the wound thereafter.

Wound irrigation – this is not always necessary; in the event of a traumatic wound whereby a wound may be contaminated with debris and bacteria, it may be essential to irrigate the wound thoroughly to rid the wound of contaminants. Care must be taken in the event of underlying bone fractures or exposed tendons, and the patient may necessitate a transfer to a minor injuries or accident and emergency department for specialised care and treatment.

In most wound cases, however, simple tap water irrigation will rid the wound of more contaminants and bacteria than will be applied to the wound from the non-sterile solution. In cases where the wound is a new surgical wound, if there is an underlying fracture, or if the patient's general health is compromised, it is advisable to use sterile saline to irrigate the wound.

The frequency of wound irrigation will depend on the clinical findings of the wound; for example, if there is any loose debris that can be removed by irrigation; if the wound is infected, or if there are high levels of wound exudate that make it more probable than not the wound will become infected, then it is advisable to thoroughly irrigate the wound to reduce (but not eliminate) the bacterial levels on the wound, which will return the pH levels of the wound to within normal range over time. Once the exudate levels reduce to a 'moist' level and providing there is no loose debris on the wound, then once weekly irrigation can be carried out to maintain control over the bacterial levels that will inevitably multiply over time if irrigation did not occur at all. Although irrigation will not remove all bacterium, it will reduce the numbers on the wound bed. Without such irrigation, numbers will simply increase until the wound becomes critically colonised and healing is unable to progress.

It must however be kept in mind that unnecessary irrigation will simply delay wound healing as brand new vulnerable granulation or epithelial cells can be easily damaged or washed away. Therefore, a fine balance must be achieved.

When irrigating a wound it is vital that gauze swabs are not used and that the irrigating fluid is poured over the wound instead. Using gauze simply causes trauma and pain on wound contact and simply spreads the bacteria around the wound without removal.

Wound swabs – it is general practice that a wound swab is taken when two or more clinical signs of infection are present in order to assist in identifying the causative bacterium. There is little benefit in taking a wound swab when the wound is progressing towards healing as the bacteria living on the wound are clearly insufficient to hinder the healing rates. With good irrigation at timely intervals and the use of appropriate dressings, the wound should continue to progress providing all other holistic factors influencing the healing rates are also addressed.

In the event that a wound swab is obtained, the results will depend on what part of the wound the swab has made contact with; as bacteria live in colonies it is possible that the causative bacteria may not make contact with the swab, so inappropriate antibiotics are often prescribed. Similarly, any wound will be contaminated or colonized with bacteria, so any swab taken from even a healthy non-infected wound will grow microbes. Therefore, care must be taken to avoid unnecessary use of antibiotics that could lead to bacterial resistance that could place the patient at risk of prolonged healing rates.

Aseptic technique – the principles of aseptic technique must be applied when dealing with any wound; the use of sterile gloves is not necessary for older wounds, but gloves must be changed after removal of the old dressing, and again after wound irrigation in order to apply the new dressing. In cases where there are underlying bone fractures, a new surgical wound or if the patient is immune-compromised, then it is advisable to use sterile gloves throughout, changing them at the steps already stated.

In all circumstances, a sterile dressing must be applied to the wound from an unopened, undamaged product wrapper. Any unused dressings must be disposed of and should not be kept for future use.

Pain control – Prior to commencing with dressing changes or wound treatments, it is vital to assess the patients pain levels using an appropriate pain tool, analgesia must then be given as necessary allowing sufficient time for this to take effect before wound care is commenced. Reassessment of pain should be carried out following dressing change, and this is discussed in greater detail in another chapter.

Maintaining the above principles let us look now at the application of dressings in the following chapter.

Wound Care at a Glance, First Edition. Ian Peate and Wyn Glencross. © 2015 John Wiley & Sons, Ltd. Published 2015 by John Wiley & Sons, Ltd.
Companion website: www.ataglanceseries.com/nursing/woundcare

25 Principles of wound management II

As stated in previous chapters the aim of wound management is to achieve a 'moist' wound healing environment, with the exception of the necrotic, ischaemic wound, which must be kept dry in order to minimize the risk of gas gangrene occurring. Apart from this the only other exception to moist wound healing is with the over-granulating tissues. If the wound is too wet, it requires absorbent dressings, if it is too dry the wound needs rehydrating, either by insulating the wound so the body can donate moisture or by adding moisture using hydrating products such as hydrogels or hydrocolloids. In any event, once a wound reaches a 'moist' level it is not necessary to add moisture with hydrating products.

Care must be taken when using hydrating products and the holistic health of the patient must be considered, as to donate moisture too quickly will increase the speed of bacterial growth, thereby placing the patient at increased risk of infection. In such cases it is safer to treat a wound 'conservatively' by insulating the wound with an appropriate dressing that allows the body to donate the necessary moisture spontaneously. While this is a safer option, it is a much slower method to debride debris from a wound than if hydrating products were used, therefore risks versus benefits must be considered. Additionally, the patient's oral intake of fluids must be encouraged as the dehydrated patients wound will remain dry. Weigh up the risks versus benefits of hydrating a wound, aiming to achieve and maintain a 'moist' wound balance.

Typical care plan to manage wound moisture levels

This should detail the site of the wound and the aim of the care plan; how a wound will be managed; as a minimum it should describe the necessary steps required such as when to irrigate a wound, include the dressing type(s), frequency of dressing changes and when the wound ought to be reassessed.

A crucial aspect of maintaining a moist wound environment is the frequency of dressing changes; if a dressing becomes saturated the moisture that will be produced by the wound will have nowhere to go so will macerate the surrounding skin. If a wound is very wet it may require several dressing changes in a day; if a wound is very dry, it may not need changing very often. The nurse must therefore observe the dressing for signs of exudate strike-through. It is not advisable to leave a dressing *in situ* for longer than 7 days even if there is no strike-through visible.

Below is a typical Wound Management Care Plan that would be suitable for most wounds. Please be aware that all deeper wounds or cavity/sinus wounds will require filling with a suitable dressing (not a hydrogel). If a hydrofibre or an alginate is placed directly on any wound bed this will create a moist environment only if it is covered with a modern insulating dressing, otherwise it will dehydrate and adhere to the wound bed as the moisture is evaporated through a non-insulating dressing:

Wound Management Care Plan example

1 Irrigate the wound daily if the wound is infected; if not infected irrigate at least once a week, and more often (e.g. two or three times a week) if the wound is 'wet'. This will assist in reducing bacterial levels on the wound bed. Do not touch the wound bed or use swabs to cleanse the wound bed when irrigating as this will cause trauma and delayed wound healing. Unnecessary irrigation will delay healing.
2 Gently pat dry the surrounding skin; do not touch the wound bed.
3 Apply a primary dressing depending on the clinical findings as follows:
   (a) if the wound is moist or wet, use a hydrofibre or an alginate directly on the wound bed;
   (b) if the wound is infected use an antimicrobial dressing on the wound bed until the infection resolves;
   (c) if the wound is dry, consider using a hydrating product (only after risks versus benefits have been considered and found to be appropriate).
4 Apply a moisture barrier to the peri-wound skin; allow it to dry.
5 Cover the above with an appropriate secondary dressing as follows:
   (a) if the wound is wet use an absorbent foam dressing;
   (b) if the wound is moist use an absorbent foam dressing or a hydrocolloid, based on assessment of risk versus benefits;
   (c) if the wound is dry and the patient is fit and healthy with no ischaemia of the wound, a hydrating product can be used;
   (d) if the wound is dry and the risks of using hydrating products outweigh the benefits, the debridement/rehydrating process can be stimulated by moistening about 10% of the alginate or hydrofibre dressing before applying it to the wound, then cover it with either a foam (for a longer wear time) or a film dressing.
6 Observe the dressing for signs of exudate strike-through.
7 Change the dressing immediately exudate strike-through appears and repeat the above process. This will avoid maceration of the peri-wound skin and granulation tissue and will maintain a moist environment.
8 Record each dressing changes on the Care Plan Evaluation noting any concerns/changes in the wound. If necessary, reassess the wound.
9 Reassess the wound weekly, fortnightly or monthly (depending on the care setting and speed of healing) and record the findings on the Wound Assessment Chart (Figure 20.1).
10 REMEMBER:

RISKS versus BENEFITS ⚖ MOISTURE BALANCE

Wound Care at a Glance, First Edition. Ian Peate and Wyn Glencross. © 2015 John Wiley & Sons, Ltd. Published 2015 by John Wiley & Sons, Ltd.
Companion website: www.ataglanceseries.com/nursing/woundcare.

26 Managing wound exudate

Figure 26.1   A moist/damp environment

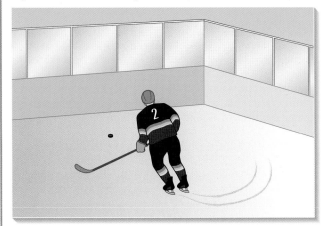

Figure 26.2   A moist/damp wound environment

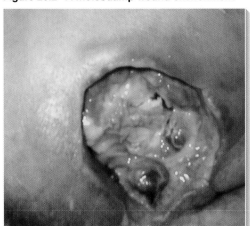

Figure 26.3   A dry environment

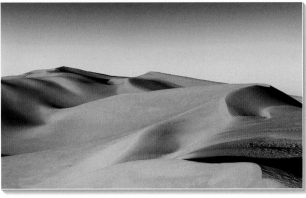

Source: iStock © hadynyah.

Figure 26.4   A dry wound environment

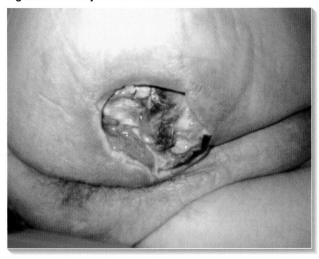

Figure 26.5   A wet environment

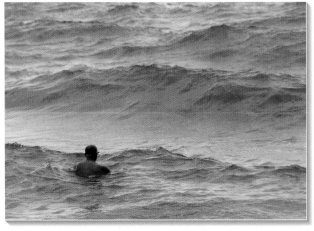

Source: iStock © cenix.

Figure 26.6   A wet wound environment

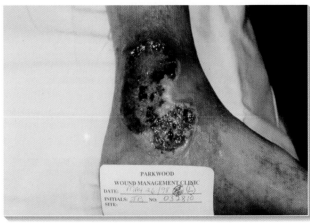

Source: Keast et al 2008, figure 9, S15. Reproduced with permission of Wiley & Sons Ltd.

Wound Care at a Glance, First Edition. Ian Peate and Wyn Glencross. © 2015 John Wiley & Sons, Ltd. Published 2015 by John Wiley & Sons, Ltd.
Companion website: www.ataglanceseries.com/nursing/woundcare

Moist wound healing

A wound will heal five times faster in a moist environment when compared to healing rates in a dry environment. By creating a moist wound environment it will facilitate all four phases of wound healing, while minimizing the growth of bacteria on the wound bed, thereby reducing the risk of wound infection.

During the healing phase, a moist wound will decrease the intensity and duration of the inflammatory response, while trapping enzymes produced within the wound bed throughout the healing process. These enzymes facilitate autolytic debridement, which prevents the build-up of debris on a wound bed (e.g. slough, necrosis and eschar). This therefore allows for easier and quicker migration of granulation and epithelial cells across the wound bed that would otherwise be obstructed by these barriers if the wound was dry and covered with debris. A moist wound will preserve the growth factors that are produced within the wound fluid, which assist with faster healing times. A moist wound will increase collagen synthesis and angiogenesis, and wound contraction will occur much quicker, thereby making for a more favourable cosmetic result during the maturation phase of wound healing. Throughout this process, bacteria will find it much more difficult to multiply in a moist wound environment as they favour either wet or dry environments depending on whether they are aerobic or anaerobic bacteria. A moist wound is therefore not favourable to either type of bacteria and less likely to become infected.

It is not possible to measure the amount of exudate present on a wound, or to specify the optimum amount to achieve the above benefits. However, it is possible to say that in most cases we want a 'moist' wound as opposed to a 'wet' or a 'dry' wound. So how do we describe a moist wound? The following analogy may assist practitioners to recognize when a wound is moist, wet or dry, which can occur even when debris is present on the wound bed (i.e. necrosis, slough or eschar).

If you were to fall into a swimming pool, it would not matter how large or small that swimming pool is, you would be saturated. If on the other hand you sat in the sand in the Sahara Desert, you would be totally dry due to the absence of any moisture, whereas if you sat on an ice rink, you would be neither saturated nor dry, and instead you would be 'damp' or 'moist'. It is the 'ice rink', damp environment that is equivalent to the optimum 'moist' wound environment that we are aiming to achieve in wound management (Figures 26.1, 26.3 and 26.5).

Let us now convert this analogy to the wet, dry or moist wound.

The wet wound (Figure 26.6)

This wound will require frequent dressing changes due to saturation from excessive amounts of wound exudate (the volume of which is irrelevant as it is either wet or it isn't). There will often be visible exudate strike-through (staining) on the outer dressing as the dressing reaches its maximum absorbing ability. The moisture will then be absorbed by the peri-wound skin, causing maceration (water logging), which is white or silver in colour and may be wrinkly in appearance. If bacterial levels are high as it often is in wet environments, the pH levels will alter the exudate to a more acidic level that causes excoriation (burning) to the peri-wound skin, which will be red in appearance. On dressing removal the exudate often run off the wound.

The wet wound will destroy epithelial and granulation cells, and will dilute the growth factors thereby stopping the wound from healing altogether in most cases. Infected wounds will usually become wet and exudate levels will increase as bacterial levels increase.

The dry wound (Figure 26.4)

This wound is mostly dry and crusty and will have no sheen to it. There may be small patches of moisture present; however, it will be considered a dry wound if the majority produces little or no exudate. The dressing will be dry, and can often adhere to the wound (especially if a wrong dressing is selected). The patient often complains of a 'tightness' or pain on or around the wound. Any erythema (redness) around the wound is usually attributed to another cause such as infection, the inflammatory response or the effects of pressure rather than from excoriation, and will therefore require further assessment.

It is difficult for granulation and epithelial cells to migrate across the dry wound bed as the cells have to burrow under the dry debris. As a result of the obstruction migrating cells are easily damaged and in doing so will delay the healing process.

The moist wound (Figure 26.2)

This wound will appear 'damp' and will glisten with moisture although no moisture appears to drip from the wound. There will be no evidence of maceration or excoriation (unless from some other cause as previously stated) as exudate levels are managed adequately in the dressing, which is changed immediately any exudate strike-through appears. On average this dressing will require changing two or three times per week, and sometimes once weekly, depending on the size of the wound.

It is unusual for a moist wound to become infected providing these moisture levels are maintained. In the event that an infection does occur, it will no longer be a moist wound and will become a wet one instead.

Managing wound exudate

The optimum moist environment makes for faster healing rates as previously described. In order to achieve this it is vital that the most appropriate dressing is selected in the first instance, and timely dressing changes are carried out in the second. Dressing changes must be dictated by the levels of exudate (i.e. by evidence of strike-through) rather than an estimate of time (e.g. change every 3 days).

27 Generic wound products: mode of action

Table 27.1 A summary of different types of dressings

Generic dressing type	Common brands in each category	Indications	Contraindications	Cautions	Type of wound
Hydrocolloids	Granulfex Duoderm Hydrocoll Comfeel	Dry or low exuding wounds	Heavily exuding (wet) wounds Infected wounds Any risk of gas gangrene	Diabetic foot ulcers	Pressure ulcers Leg ulcers Surgical wounds Dehisced wounds Traumatic wounds Ruptured blisters
Foams (adhesive or non-adhesive)	Biatain Lyofoam Allevyn	Moist, moderate or heavily exuding wounds (i.e. moist to wet)	None	Sensitivities Avoid direct applications to dry wounds (unless that is the aim – discussed in other chapters) Avoid direct contact with intact skin as far as possible to prevent dehydration	All wound types
Film	Hydrofilm C-View Tegaderm Opsite	On fragile, vulnerable skin with no exudate, or on low exuding wounds if an alginate or hydrofibre is applied to the wound first	None	None	Superficial wounds of all types and on vulnerable skin or scar tissue
Alginates	Sorbsan Kaltostat	For all wounds with any level of moisture. Can be moistened by 20% if the wound is dry	None	Sensitivities Must be covered with an insulating dressing	All wound types Not suitable if the wound is to be completely dried out as it will remain moist
Hydrofibre	Aquacel (plain)	For all wounds with any level of moisture. Can be moistened by 20% if the wound is dry	None	Sensitivities Must be covered with an insulating dressing	All wound types Not suitable if the wound is to be completely dried out as it will remain moist
Hydrogel/Hydrogel sheet	Actiform Cool (sheet) Intrasite (gel and sheet) Nu-gel (gel) Aquagel (gel)	For dry or very low exuding wounds	Heavily exuding (wet) wounds Infected wounds Any risk of gas gangrene	Diabetic foot ulcers	All wound types
Non-adherent	Silicone or knitted fabrics (N/A) Mepitel Urgotulle	To prevent dressings adhering to a wound	None	May not achieve the aim of a moist wound healing environment	All wound types
Other dressing types	Absorbent pad, e.g. Kerramax, Eclipse Surgipads, Gamgee, gauze, dressing pads	With the exception of highly absorbent pads, there is very minimal place for this type of dressing in modern wound care	Not advisable for open wounds unless for exudate management of non-healing wounds	Will not insulate a wound so will have a tendency to dry a wound out, causing adherence. Some Gamgees are treated with bleach	Not recommended on any wound types, except wet, non-healing wounds such as leg ulcers, until such time the cause of exudate levels are addressed and levels reduce

Wound Care at a Glance, First Edition. Ian Peate and Wyn Glencross. © 2015 John Wiley & Sons, Ltd. Published 2015 by John Wiley & Sons, Ltd.
Companion website: www.ataglanceseries.com/nursing/woundcare

Wound products

It is essential that any product chosen for use on a wound is selected on the basis of the clinical assessment of the wound and the holistic assessment of the patient and in accordance with the aims that the nurse is trying to achieve.

It is essential that the products used on a wound are prescribed; however, because most nurses are not qualified to prescribe, it is common for dressings to be selected from a 'Dressings Formulary'. This is a list of wound care dressing products that have been scrutinized and approved by an organization for use on wounds, and therefore negates the need for each and every product on that formulary to be prescribed. The nurse will therefore be supported legally if she/he selects a product from a formulary providing she/he had used it for the purposes it is intended.

Let us now consider typical generic products that would be found on a dressing's formulary; their mode of action; when to use the and when they are contraindicated on wounds (Table 27.1).

Hydrocolloids – these are hydrating products that can be used on dry wounds with little or no moisture in order to raise the exudate levels to a moist environment. They must be changed immediately there is evidence of strike-through in order to avoid saturation, and therefore maceration or excoriation that could quickly lead to infection. Once the wound had reached the optimum 'moist' level consideration must be given to the wear time of this dressing and whether or not it remains appropriate, as it will then require more frequent dressing changes if its use continues. This product is an 'insulating' product meaning that it maintains body temperature on the wound bed, and can be used alone as the primary dressing or as a secondary dressing with alginates or hydrofibres underneath. Contraindications are listed in Table 27.1 and discussed in other chapters.

Foams – these are absorbent dressings intended to reduce exudate levels. However these products if used alone could potentially dry the wound out completely, as it will absorb exudate faster than the body can produce it. In order to avoid drying out alginates or hydrofibres can be used underneath to maintain a moist environment. They are insulating dressings, thereby maintaining body temperature on the wound. Contraindications are listed in Table 27.1 and discussed in other chapters.

Films – these products neither absorb moisture nor hydrate wounds. Used on their own they can only be used on vulnerable but unbroken skin (e.g. a Grade 1 pressure damage, areas vulnerable to friction, or on healed wounds that require some protection for a while). It can be used with either an alginate or a hydrofibre placed underneath and together this combination can be used on low to moderate exuding wounds. Films will insulate the wound thereby maintaining body temperature.

Alginates – these are absorbent primary dressings that require one of the aforementioned insulating secondary dressings applied over them. Failure to 'insulate' this type of dressing will cause it to dry and adhere to the wound bed, thereby causing trauma on removal. This type of dressing is required for deeper wounds in order to 'fill' them to skin level. They can also be applied to shallower wounds in order to assist with maintaining a 'moist' wound, and to increase the absorbency and therefore the wear time of the dressing.

Hydrofibre – this is an absorbent primary dressing that also maintains a moist wound environment if an insulating primary dressing is applied over it. It is used in the same way that an Alginate is used, however it is considered by some as having the additional benefit of trapping bacteria as it absorbs wound exudate.

Hydrogels/hydrogel sheets – these are hydrating products intended to raise the moisture levels of a dry wound to 'moist'. Hydrogels consist of approximately 20% polysaccharides and 80% water thereby producing a watery gel. Hydrogel sheets consist of approximately 20% water and 80% polysaccharides, so makes for a thicker consistency thereby forming a sheet. A gel sheet will absorb some moisture within the polysaccharides, but the liquid gel won't absorb anything. Care must be taken when selecting a secondary dressing, as to apply a liquid gel to a wound covered by a foam for example will negate the effects intended by the gel as it is absorbed into the dressing.

Non-adherent – these are dressings that don't insulate the wound, hydrate nor absorb moisture and are commonly used for superficial wounds under other dressing types to prevent them from adhering to the wound. Many wound experts consider these dressing types have little usefulness in wound care and are therefore most frequently used with vacuum-assisted closure treatments (topical negative pressure) and will be discussed later.

Other dressing types – this category includes dressing types specifically designed to provide combinations of the above dressing types for example a combination of a hydrofibre and a hydrocolloid. Alternatively, such dressings as highly absorbent pads, Gamgee, dressing pads, and other common products that are selected for their cost-effectiveness, or when the aims of the wound is to manage wound exudate when there is no prospect of a wound healing based on underlying factors. Many experts consider that the use of these products is limited due to their lack of wound insulation.

Antimicrobials – there currently are three main categories of antimicrobial dressings; silver, honey and iodine impregnated dressings. Honey and Iodine also comes in a paste or an ointment that is often applied to wounds under appropriate dressings. Selection of a particular antimicrobial will depend on the products available to the nurse on the dressing's formulary, and based on holistic and wound assessment. Antimicrobials will be discussed in greater detail in later chapters.

Conclusion

Dressing selection will depend on many things and it is important that the nurse has a sound knowledge of each dressing type available to them and the dressing's mode of action. It is important that the nurse responsible for wound care is fully aware of the indications and the contraindications for use in order to apply a dressing's formulary appropriately. Inappropriate selection can cause harm to the patient.

28 Choosing a wound care product

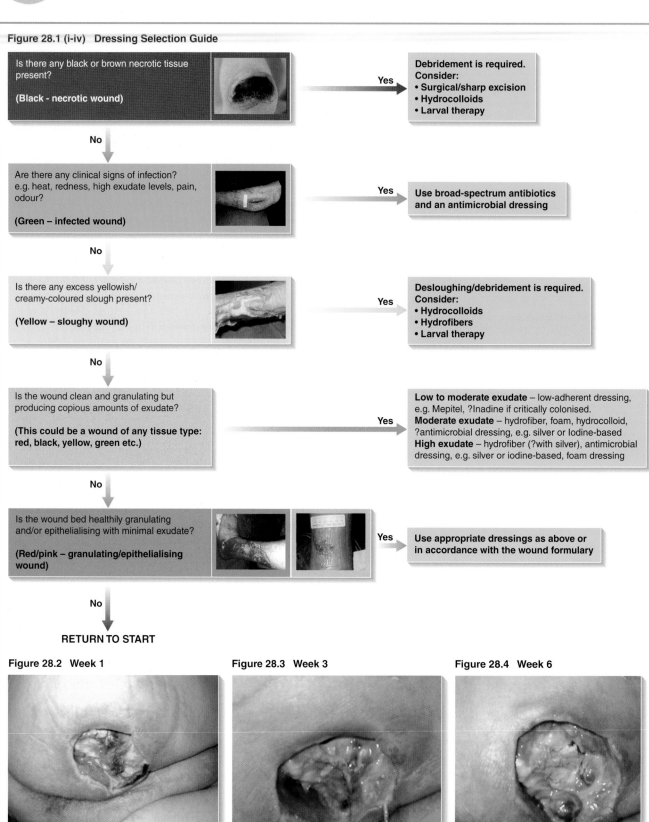

Figure 28.1 (i-iv) Dressing Selection Guide

| Is there any black or brown necrotic tissue present?

(Black - necrotic wound) | **Yes →** | **Debridement is required.
Consider:**
• Surgical/sharp excision
• Hydrocolloids
• Larval therapy |

No ↓

| Are there any clinical signs of infection?
e.g. heat, redness, high exudate levels, pain, odour?

(Green – infected wound) | **Yes →** | **Use broad-spectrum antibiotics and an antimicrobial dressing** |

No ↓

| Is there any excess yellowish/creamy-coloured slough present?

(Yellow – sloughy wound) | **Yes →** | **Desloughing/debridement is required.
Consider:**
• Hydrocolloids
• Hydrofibers
• Larval therapy |

No ↓

| Is the wound clean and granulating but producing copious amounts of exudate?

(This could be a wound of any tissue type: red, black, yellow, green etc.) | **Yes →** | **Low to moderate exudate** – low-adherent dressing, e.g. Mepitel, ?Inadine if critically colonised.
Moderate exudate – hydrofiber, foam, hydrocolloid, ?antimicrobial dressing, e.g. silver or Iodine-based
High exudate – hydrofiber (?with silver), antimicrobial dressing, e.g. silver or iodine-based, foam dressing |

No ↓

| Is the wound bed healthily granulating and/or epithelialising with minimal exudate?

(Red/pink – granulating/epithelialising wound) | **Yes →** | **Use appropriate dressings as above or in accordance with the wound formulary** |

No ↓

RETURN TO START

Figure 28.2 Week 1   Figure 28.3 Week 3   Figure 28.4 Week 6

Wound Care at a Glance, First Edition. Ian Peate and Wyn Glencross. © 2015 John Wiley & Sons, Ltd. Published 2015 by John Wiley & Sons, Ltd.
Companion website: www.ataglanceseries.com/nursing/woundcare

Aims in wound care

The aim in wound management is to achieve a 'moist' wound-healing environment in most cases (exceptions to moist healing will be discussed in later chapters). Moist healing can be achieved by the application of modern wound dressings, accompanied by timely dressing changes to prevent saturation. If this moisture level is achieved this will assist with the preparation of the wound bed so that it will heal as promptly as it possibly can.

As part of this process it is important to assess the wound in detail in order to (a) ensure the most appropriate product/treatment is selected and (b) to devise an appropriate plan of care for the ongoing management and monitoring of the wound. Although there are many aspects to consider when assessing a wound, many nurses utilize a framework known as TIME in order to systematically consider relevant issues before applying a treatment, as follows:

Tissue, Infection, Moisture, Edge (TIME)

Tissue – the nurse makes note of the tissue type on the wound bed. Any tissue that may require removal could inlcude dead and devitalized tissue such as necrosis, or unwanted debris such as slough, dead skin or foreign bodies, all of which can inhibit healing rates while creating a harbour for bacterial growth. Consideration must be given to the most appropriate method to remove unwanted tissue. This could be achieved by autolytic debridement, by the use of larval therapy (maggots), by sharp debridement by a nurse trained in the technique, or by surgical debridement under anaesthetic by a surgeon.

Infection – the nurse observes the wound and surrounding skin and tissues for any signs of infection. High levels of bacteria will usually produce high levels of exudate so could be the only indication that bacterial levels on a wound is high. A wet wound in the absence of two or more clinical signs of infection would be regarded as heavily (or critically) colonized wound and not infected. Treatment choice will depend on whether or not an infection has been clinically identified.

Moisture – moisture levels on a wound can vary from light to heavy within hours for a variety of reasons (e.g. bacteria levels; leaking oedema; hydrating products). The nurse must therefore continually assess the moisture levels oozing from a wound in order to select the most appropriate dressing product to manage it. Failure to do so will allow excess moisture onto the wound and surrounding tissues, which will cause maceration thereby hindering healing while creating an optimum environment for rapid bacterial growth thereby increasing the risk of infection.

Edge – the nurse must observe the edges of the wound for signs of healing (by granulation, epithelialization and wound shrinkage by maturation), as well as for signs of infection and/or damage to surrounding tissues caused by maceration or excoriation from poorly contained moisture levels, or from damage or allergy to products used. Any untoward signs will determine what product is or is not to be used on a wound.

Dressing selection guide

Once the nurse has assessed the wound and surrounding skin/tissues, it is essential that she/he records this on a Wound Assessment Chart. These findings in conjunction with the findings on holistic assessment of the patient will enable the nurse to identify the aims of care required to remove unwanted tissue (if any); avoid the production of unwanted tissue; promote healing while eradicating/preventing infection and/or damage to healthy tissues by appropriately managing exudate levels, all of which must be included in a care plan that will direct others on the management of the wound to achieve these aims.

The Dressing Selection Guide shown in Figure 28.1 will assist the nurse in selecting the most appropriate product once the patient and his/her wound has been fully assessed, by considering the clinical findings to reach the most appropriate treatment option.

Case study

Mr Joe Bloggs is an 83-year-old multiple sclerosis patient who sustained a Grade 4 pressure ulcer while an inpatient undergoing a prostatectomy. He has no other medical history, he is mentally competent, communicates verbally, has no allergies, is fully dependent on others for all activities of daily living. He has a normal range body mass index and is otherwise reasonably healthy with good immunity. His wound is sited over the right ischial tuberosity (the bones we sit on). Using TIME, an assessment of the wound shown in Figure 28.2 divulges the following clinical findings:

T – tissue on the wound bed consists of approximately 85% slough and 15% healthy granulation tissue.

I – There is no evidence of infection (no surrounding erythema, pus, dry to minimal exudate, no malodour or pain and no friable wound bed)

M – Moisture levels are minimal (confirmed by the absence of maceration or excoriation to the surrounding skin), and the dressing was not saturated on removal after 6 days.

E – Edges of the wound were healthy: no maceration, excoriation, trauma or allergic reactions.

Using the dressing selection guide

Based on the holistic and wound findings, effective pressure relief was provided and it was agreed that the patients health and immunity was sufficient to withstand active autolytic debridement (discussed later) by way of hydrocolloids rather than by passive autolytic debridement (also discussed later) or surgical intervention. Hydrocolloids were stopped once the wound had become moist (Figure 28.3), and passive autolytic debridement was adopted thereafter until the wound was fully healed. Figure 28.4 shows the wound almost fully debrided, but with a significantly shallower wound depth, which came about by allowing granulation tissue to fill the wound in the moist environment that was maintained throughout. The surrounding skin was healthy throughout and there were no wound infection events during the process.

Use of topical antimicrobials and antibiotics

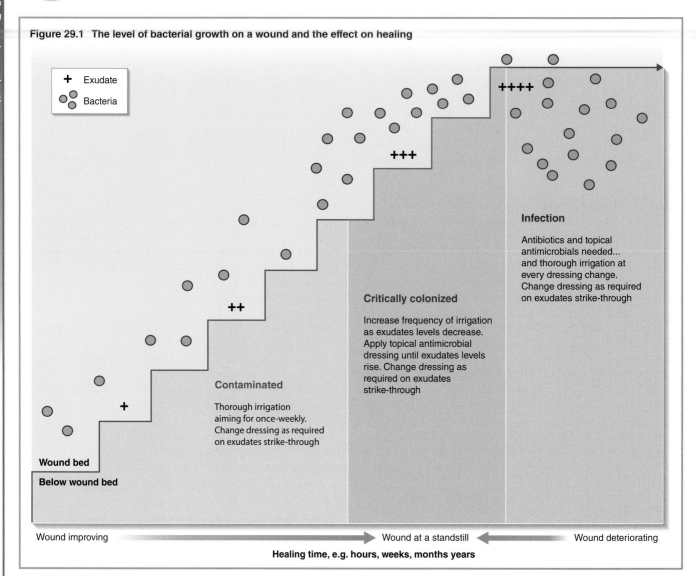

Figure 29.1 The level of bacterial growth on a wound and the effect on healing

Legend:
+ Exudate
Bacteria

Contaminated

Thorough irrigation aiming for once-weekly. Change dressing as required on exudates strike-through

Critically colonized

Increase frequency of irrigation as exudates levels decrease. Apply topical antimicrobial dressing until exudates levels rise. Change dressing as required on exudates strike-through

Infection

Antibiotics and topical antimicrobials needed... and thorough irrigation at every dressing change. Change dressing as required on exudates strike-through

Wound bed
Below wound bed

Wound improving — Wound at a standstill — Wound deteriorating

Healing time, e.g. hours, weeks, months years

Wound Care at a Glance, First Edition. Ian Peate and Wyn Glencross. © 2015 John Wiley & Sons, Ltd. Published 2015 by John Wiley & Sons, Ltd.
Companion website: www.ataglanceseries.com/nursing/woundcare

Spreading infection at the wound site requires treatment with systemic antibiotics. Additionally, a topical antimicrobial dressing ought to be applied to the wound bed to assist in reducing bacterial levels on the wound, which will reduce the risk of reinfection once systemic antibiotics have eliminated the infection under the wound bed.

Topical antimicrobials, while reducing the bacterial bio-burden on the wound bed, will not eliminate a spreading infection. Infection risk can be reduced if bacterial levels on the wound are kept to a minimum, as it is most commonly the high number of bacteria (of any species) living on the wound bed rather than specific species that is important in the treatment of most infections. Control of bacterial growth can be better achieved by maintaining a 'moist' wound-healing environment; by thorough irrigation of the wound bed at appropriate intervals; and by the use of topical antimicrobial dressings and other wound treatment products when they are required. Figure 29.1 gives guidance on when to use each of these methods of control.

Common antimicrobials

At the time of writing, there are three main types of antimicrobial products available. The following will discuss the pros and cons of each product. Selection will depend on the findings of a holistic and wound assessment and the products that are accessible to the health professional, who would usually select a product from a Wound Dressing Formulary agreed within their organization.

Honey and honey-impregnated dressings

Medical grade honey has antimicrobial and anti-inflammatory properties and can be used for acute or chronic wounds. Honey has osmotic properties that produce an environment that promotes autolytic debridement (i.e. the removal of debris on the wound bed). As it kills and reduces bacterial levels so in turn is malodour reduced. It is a reasonably cost-effective product and is effective on a large number of bacterial species.

The disadvantages of using honey are that not all bacteria are eradicated with honey, and indeed some bacteria are known to thrive on the presence of sugar found in the honey. As the honey has an osmotic affect, the end product will be H_2O (water), which could make for a wet wound, which would then be conducive for rapid bacterial growth, and as there is no sustained release of antimicrobial product, the wet environment could lead to reinfection. It is therefore vital that the dressing is closely observed for exudate strike-through (staining on the outer dressing) and that it is changed before it becomes saturated. The increased dressing changes and risk of reinfection could negate any savings made on using this cheaper antimicrobial. And finally, care must be taken when using this product on patients who are diabetics, and regular blood sugar checks must be made. Care must also be taken when using the product on those with known hypersensitivities to bee stings.

Iodine and iodine-impregnated dressings

This product is commonly chosen as a first-line antimicrobial because it is cheap to purchase. The two main types of iodine are discussed below.

1 Cadexomer iodine is placed in ointments and pastes. This enables the release of free iodine when exposed to wound exudate. This serves as an antiseptic on the wound surface. It can absorb exudate and aid desloughing of wound debris. Common products in this category are Iodoflex and Iodosorb. Disadvantages are that there is a known (and increasing) bacterial resistance; systemic absorption of iodine can occur if applied to a large wound or used for prolonged periods and should therefore only be used in accordance with directions in the BNF. It is contraindicated for pregnant and breast-feeding women, for thyroid conditions and those who are prescribed lithium. As it is absorbed it is difficult to achieve a sustained release of antimicrobial, which means that reinfection can easily occur.

2 Povidone iodine is impregnated into a knitted viscose dressing incorporated in a hydrophilic polyethylene glycol base that facilitates diffusion of the iodine onto the wound bed. It has a wide spectrum of antimicrobial activity; however, this is rapidly deactivated on contact with wound exudate. An example that is commonly used is Inadine. Disadvantages of this product are that it is difficult to achieve a sustained release of antimicrobials as the iodine is deactivated with wound exudate; therefore, reinfection can easily occur.

Silver-impregnated dressings

Silver has a broad spectrum of antimicrobial activity and has, to date, no known bacterial resistance. The volume of wound exudate must be considered when choosing a silver dressing. There are no known contraindications for silver dressings, with the exception of those containing silver sulphadiazine, which are silver salts impregnated into a dressing that may be absorbed, causing blood disorders and skin discolouration. Other types of silver dressing can be of the metallic or ionic silver types, neither of which is absorbed so there are no contraindications for their use. People with an allergy to metallic silver may be at risk of a reaction; however, providing the dressing containing metallic silver is not in contact with the skin and only with wound exudate, the metal aspect will be converted to ionic silver in a chemical reaction with the exudate. To date there is no known allergy to ionic silver, and it is not absorbed. Disadvantages of silver products are the cost. However, if they are chosen carefully, they can be left *in situ* on the wound for a number of days, thereby changing only the outer dressing and reducing costs.

Topical antibiotics must be avoided unless directed by a specialist as the antibiotic is usually impregnated into a gel or a cream; as the infected wound will usually be a 'wet' wound the antibiotic is diluted and absorbed into the dressing, so there is no sustained release of antibiotic. This leads to bacterial resistance to that antibiotic.

30 Application of lotions, creams, emollients and ointments

Figure 30.1 The Dermol range of emollients

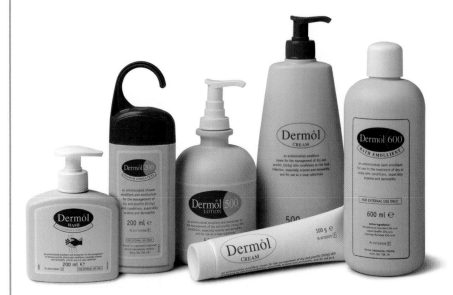

Source: Dermal Laboratories Ltd. Reproduced with permission of Dermal Laboratories Ltd.

Figure 30.2 Epaderm cream, which is used to manage skin conditions such as eczema and psoriasis

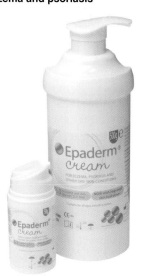

Source: Mölnlycke Health Care. Reproduced with permission of Mölnlycke Health Care.

Figure 30.3 The Cavilon range of barrier products, which act to protect the skin from excess moisture, e.g. from body fluids

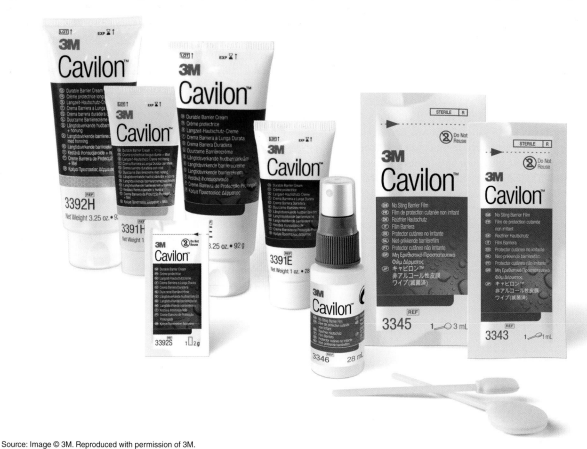

Source: Image © 3M. Reproduced with permission of 3M.

Wound Care at a Glance, First Edition. Ian Peate and Wyn Glencross. © 2015 John Wiley & Sons, Ltd. Published 2015 by John Wiley & Sons, Ltd.
Companion website: www.ataglanceseries.com/nursing/woundcare

Appropriate and effective skin care is a vital part of maintaining tissue viability, particularly as we age because of slower cell regeneration. It is particularly important to care for the skin in order to protect it from moisture damage. Moisture damage can occur from sweating, particularly on skin folds, from incontinence of urine and faeces, and around peri-wound skin from wound exudate.

The skin is affected by external conditions such as low humidity, by excessive bathing using soaps and other products that can strip it of natural oils (sebum) causing it to dry. Smoking habits, sun exposure, poor levels of hydration and poor nutrition can further impact on skin integrity.

The skin's natural moisturiser and water barrier comes from sebum; as we age the sebum production reduces so our skin becomes drier and/or more prone to moisture damage. Dry skin can lead to itching, cracking, scaling and inflammation, thereby resulting in breaches of the skin through which bacteria can invade, causing skin infection (cellulitis). Excess moisture on the skin can cause excoriation or maceration, which again breaches this protective layer thereby increasing the risk of cellulitis.

This chapter will focus on the types of products that are available that can enhance the quality and integrity of the skin, thereby going some way to protect it from the effects of day to day living.

Moisturisers

Moisturisers are the most effective way of substituting the loss and/or the reduction of sebum, as they help restore the barrier function of the epidermis. Indeed, they are an essential aspect of daily skin care as they slow the loss of skin moisture through evaporation. They maintain skin suppleness, prevent drying and cracking, while improving the appearance of the skin.

Moisturisers should ideally be applied twice daily to intact skin and should not be applied between toes or in skin folds as this will increase the risk of fungal infections in these areas. Typically moisturisers are made up of water and petroleum. Un-perfumed and alcohol-free products are most beneficial to avoid skin irritation or reactions.

Ointments, creams and lotions

Ointments – These products are similar to moisturisers in that they produce a protective layer over the skin. Ointments are typically thicker in consistency than moisturisers and are primarily made from water and oils (e.g. lanolin, which can cause skin reactions in some people).

Creams and lotions – these are thinner in consistency than moisturisers and ointments as they consist primarily of water. As a result they are less effective at hydrating dry skin as they require more frequent applications. They are less occlusive than moisturisers

and ointments, so are less effective at protecting from the effects of moisture.

Emollients

Emollients are also known as moisturisers. They can be used to wash the skin and they can be applied directly to the skin as with other moisturisers (e.g. Dermol range, Figure 30.1). Emollients are particularly useful in protecting the skin from irritants (e.g. under bandages); they are the preferred moisturiser for people with sensitive skin and for those who have eczema as they can prevent flare-ups of these conditions (e.g. Epaderm cream, Figure 30.2). These products can be purchased directly from a pharmacy and are available on prescription.

Steroid creams and ointments

These products differ from emollients and other moisturisers and are intended to be used to clear up flare-ups of skin conditions such as eczema and are not intended for regular use unless directed by a physician.

Barrier creams (Figure 30.3)

While the aforementioned products (with the exception of steroid creams and ointments) will provide an element of moisture barrier, where excess moisture exists it is advisable to use specific barrier creams. These products have the added benefit of petroleum and/or zinc oxide, which provide a greater degree of moisture barrier. Barrier creams should only be applied to intact skin.

Some barrier creams contain alcohol, which if applied to broken skin will cause stinging, so should be avoided. Similarly, the barrier creams that have a thicker consistency will cause excess friction on the skin during application and removal so should also be avoided as far as possible. Furthermore, these thicker creams are often contraindicated by incontinence pad manufacturers as they leave a film on the pad that can inhibit its absorbency ability, causing moisture to run off the pad and/or spread to wider areas of unprotected skin. These type of creams also obscure the skin making observation of the skin difficult.

Barrier sprays (Figure 30.3)

These products are useful for use on superficial skin breaks and rashes; for example on continence lesions, rashes, and on peri-wound skin, taking care to avoid the wound itself. Sprays allow adhesive dressings to be applied to the skin, whereas barrier creams don't.

Finally

It is essential that products are chosen based on holistic assessment and that manufacturer recommendations are always adhered to.

31 Advanced technologies

Figure 31.1 VAC pump

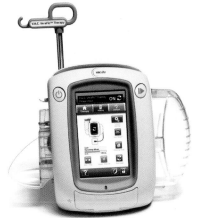

Source: KCI. Used with permission. Courtesy of KCI.

Figure 31.2 Diagram of TNP

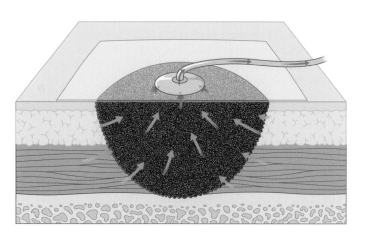

Figure 31.3 Larval therapy

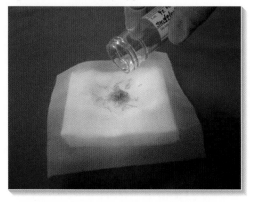

Figure 31.4 Maggots on the wound

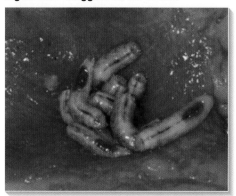

Source: The Surgical Materials Testing Laboratory. Reproduced with permission of The Surgical Materials Testing Laboratory.

Figure 31.5 Colonies of *Pseudomonas* after larval therapy

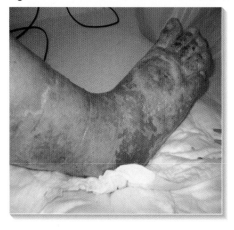

Figure 31.6 Versajet

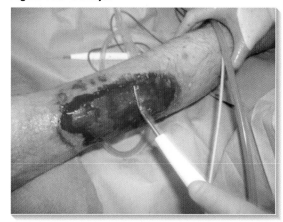

Wound Care at a Glance, First Edition. Ian Peate and Wyn Glencross. © 2015 John Wiley & Sons, Ltd. Published 2015 by John Wiley & Sons, Ltd.
Companion website: www.ataglanceseries.com/nursing/woundcare

Research into wound healing is progressing at significant rates and much of the work is focused around removing debris and speeding up the healing process of wounds. Additionally, scientists strive to find new ways of preventing infections; however, in some cases, ancient tried and tested methods do not appear to have been effectively surpassed to date.

This chapter is intended to give an overview of some of the technologies that are now well established and even ancient, and those that are up and coming, which may or may not be more commonly used in the future.

Topical negative pressure (TNP)

This commonly used technique is also known as vacuum-assisted closure (VAC) therapy; it is where a special dressing type is applied directly to a wound that is sealed in place with a film dressing, which is then attached by tubing to a special suction pump (Figure 31.1). When the pump is operational it then creates suction in the wound causing negative pressure (Figure 31.2). Negative pressures at 125 mmHg appears to enhance the phases of wound healing, not least because it increases the blood supply to the wound bed, while providing good exudate control and a moist wound-healing environment. Wounds treated with TNP appear to have fewer complications and have significantly faster healing rates. If the wound is likely to require long-term dressings, TNP can be more cost-effective than traditional dressings over a longer period of time. As dressings only require changing over 48 or 72 hours, this method of wound treatment can reduce nursing time, leaving the patient with greater independence, as this treatment can be suitable for patients in any setting, including in the community.

There are however disadvantages with this treatment, including having to fully debride a wound before the treatment can be commenced. This in itself can be time-consuming and costly, so the prevention of debris on a wound with good exudate management is vital to speed up the application of this therapy. Many patients report pain on dressing changes with TNP, making this treatment intolerable, particularly for those with vascular disease in their lower limbs, which is unfortunate as these wounds would benefit from the treatment due to an increased blood flow. The treatment is contraindicated for bleeding wounds, fistulas (unless approved by a specialist) and malignant wounds, and any underlying osteomyelitis (bone infection) must be treated for at least 2 weeks prior to the application of this treatment. Other disadvantages of the treatment besides cost are mechanical failures such as kinked tubing, loss of suction and the inability to achieve a good seal in the first place, especially if the wound is sited near an orifice such as the anus.

Larval (maggot) therapy (Figures 31.3 and 31.4)

Maggots have been working their magic on wounds for centuries, saving many a life during war times. They work by excreting an enzyme that then liquefies dead and devitalized tissues on a wound. The maggot then drinks this liquid, thereby removing slough and necrosis from the wound bed until it eventually reveals healthy granulation tissues. An entire limb can be removed this way if it no longer consists of living tissue. Maggots are however contraindicated on fistula wounds, and bleeding wounds.

Known affectionately as 'the world's smallest surgeon', maggots will debride a wound faster than autolytic debridement (i.e. using dressings to mimic what maggots do). Interestingly, they are known to eradicate in their gut the bacteria they take in with the wound exudate, including bacteria such as methicillin-resistant *Staphyloccocus aureus* (MRSA). However, *Pseudomonas* appears to upset the maggots, often killing large numbers, so they tend to avoid taking in this bacteria (Figure 31.5 shows a limb after one treatment of larval therapy. The limb was originally covered in slough, much of which was removed by the first treatment. The two 'blue' areas are colonies of *Pseudomonas*, which the maggots did not touch).

Versajet

This is a device rather like a high-pressure washer; it sprays sterile water at high speed onto the wound in order to evacuate and/or excise debris, bacteria and contaminants from the wound bed (Figure 31.6).

Electrical stimulation

During the process of wound healing the body has a system whereby a bioelectrical current is sent to the injured site, which enhances the healing rate of a wound (or any other traumatized tissue or bone). In some cases this electric current short circuits for some reason and the wound either fails to heal or is very slow to heal.

One of the most exciting developments in wound treatments in recent years is the use of electrostimulation in the non-healing or stagnant wound. It is thought that an external electrical current applied to the wound bed (situated within a dressing) will mimic the natural bioelectric current that appears to be absent in the non-healing wound, thereby progressing the wound through the tissue repair processes mentioned earlier in this book. This treatment then accelerates the healing rate of the wound by attracting neutrophils, increasing the growth of fibroblasts and other growth factors, promoting granulation tissue by increasing the blood flow to the wound bed, and finally by inducing epidermal cell migration. Studies have should significantly improved healing rates on otherwise non-healing wounds when this treatment has been applied.

Interestingly, electrostimulation is thought to attract macrophages to the wound bed, which reduces the risk of infection in these wound types. This in itself is a significant breakthrough and would hopefully go some way to boost an individual's immunity, even in wounds that have little prospect of healing due to a significantly reduced blood supply for example. However, while this treatment shows promise, much more research is needed in the field of electrostimulation before it becomes a treatment choice in chronic, non-healing wounds.

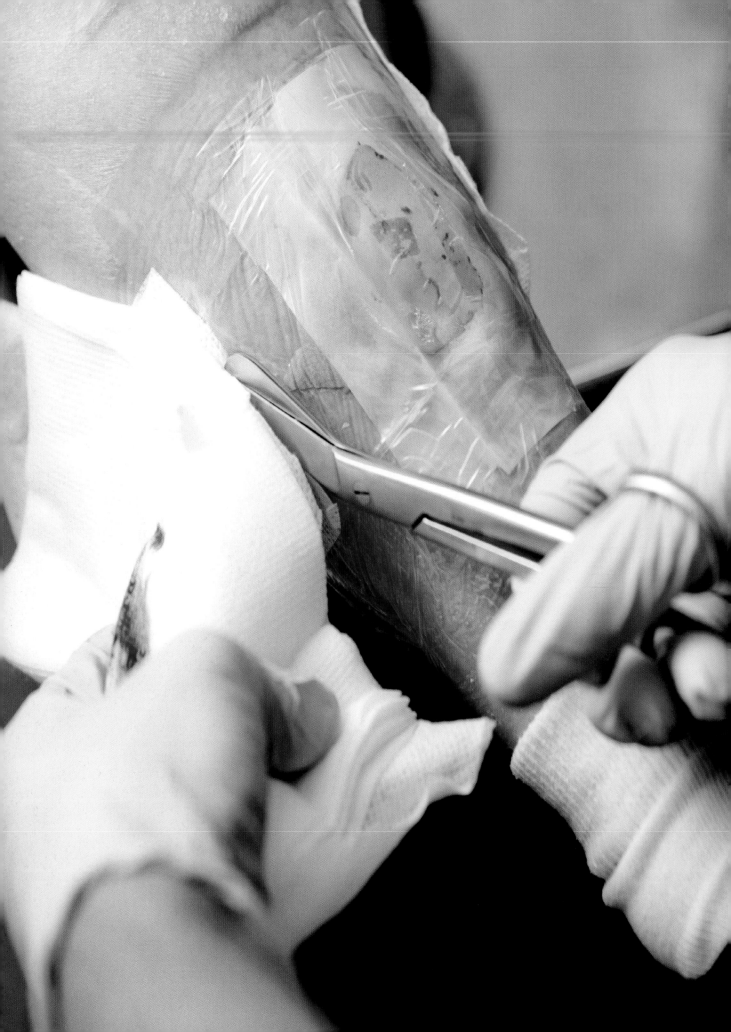

Complexities of wound care

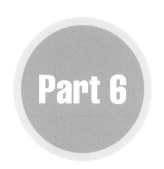

Part 6

 Visit the companion website at www.ataglanceseries.com/nursing/woundcare to test yourself on these topics.

32 Pressure redistribution equipment

Figure 32.1 A static foam mattress

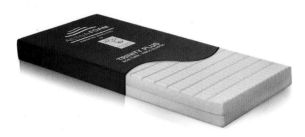

Source: Ultimate Healthcare, Frontier Medical Group. Reproduced with permission of Carl May and Steve Tetlow, Ultimate Healthcare Group

Figure 32.2 A static pressure-relieving cushion (foam)

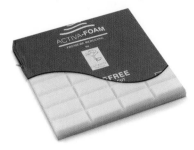

Source: Ultimate Healthcare, Frontier Medical Group. Reproduced with permission of Carl May and Steve Tetlow, Ultimate Healthcare Group

Figure 32.3 A dynamic alternating air mattress (full replacement)

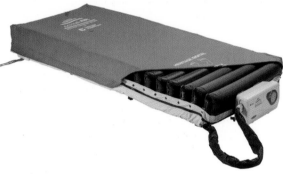

Source: Ultimate Healthcare, Frontier Medical Group. Reproduced with permission of Carl May and Steve Tetlow, Ultimate Healthcare Group

Figure 32.4 A dynamic alternating air mattress (overlay)

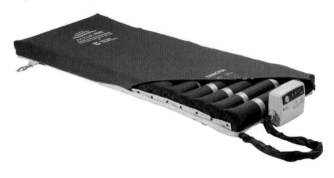

Source: Ultimate Healthcare, Frontier Medical Group. Reproduced with permission of Carl May and Steve Tetlow, Ultimate Healthcare Group

Figure 32.5 A dynamic alternating air cushion

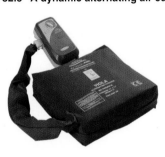

Source: Ultimate Healthcare, Frontier Medical Group. Reproduced with permission of Carl May and Steve Tetlow, Ultimate Healthcare Group

Figure 32.6 Foot Protectors (a) and supporting wedge (b)

(a)

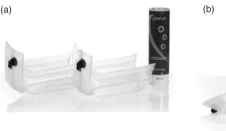

(b)

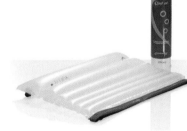

Source: Repose, Frontier Medical Group. Reproduced with permission of Matthew Clutterbuck, Frontier Medical Group

Pressure damage is caused first and foremost by prolonged, unrelieved pressure against the skin and underlying tissues. Pressure damage is exacerbated by the presence of friction and shearing, which will make the skin and underlying tissues more vulnerable to the effects of pressure. The speed at which a pressure ulcer will develop will depend on many factors that are extrinsic and intrinsic to the patient, and these must be addressed as far as possible in order to reduce the probability of a pressure ulcer developing.

The use of appropriate pressure-relieving devices is one way to deal with extrinsic factors that affect the probability of the patient developing a pressure ulcer. These devices will distribute pressure over a greater area, which means pressure ulcers will take longer to develop than they would otherwise do if the patient was not nursed on an appropriate pressure-relieving device.

Therefore, it is very important to point out that patients who are nursed on these devices will inevitably develop a pressure ulcer eventually if they are not repositioned at regular intervals, regardless of how high the specification of such devices are. These devices simply distribute pressure so that the patient can go for longer without being moved. The frequency of repositioning has been addressed elsewhere in this book.

There is a huge range of products on the market that claim to distribute pressure effectively and the cost of such devices vary widely. Selecting a device will depend on the findings on clinical judgement and on the findings of a pressure ulcer risk assessment. This chapter will give an overview of the main types of devices available, and will then discuss when each type is appropriate based on national guidelines.

National guidelines

The National Institute of Clinical Excellent (2005, 2014) and the European Pressure Ulcer Advisory Panel (2009) recommend the following devices for use under those individuals at risk of pressure damage.

1 Any patient who has a Grade 3 or 4 pressure ulcer must be nursed on a dynamic air mattress and cushion.
2 Any patient deemed to be at elevated risk must be nursed on a high-specification (e.g. viscoelastic) foam mattress and cushion, providing they have no pressure ulcers greater than Grade 2.
3 A standard foam mattress and cushion are suitable for patients who are at risk, who have no pressure ulcers and who can reposition themselves competently and independently.

Determining the level of risk must include the use of a risk assessment tool and clinical judgement, as the risk score may not reflect the clinical findings.

Pressure distribution devices
Static foam mattresses and cushions

These are available in a variety of sizes that will fit most beds and chairs (Figures 32.1 and 32.2). The standard foam mattress/cushion will mean that less pressure distribution is provided, so the patient will require more frequent repositioning than if a high-specification (viscoelastic) foam mattress/cushion was used. These mattresses are also available in bariatric sizes that will accommodate the heavier patient. It is therefore important that the patient is weighed regularly to ensure the most appropriate device is being used.

Dynamic air devices (mattresses and cushions)

These devices are called 'dynamic' due their active ability to alternate pressure from one area of the body to another, usually by alternate or every third cell deflating alternately. They can be purchased as either a full replacement mattress (Figure 32.3), as an overlay that lies over a standard or high-specification mattress (Figure 32.4) or as cushions (Figure 32.5). There is little evidence that one type is more effective than the other. The overlay however increases the overall height of the bed compared to a replacement mattress, and is an important consideration if bed rails are required to prevent a patient from rolling out of bed, in which case a full replacement mattress must be selected. These devices have weight limitations, which vary from one manufacturer to another, so it is important to monitor the patient's weight to ensure they are being nursed on an appropriate device. If a patient requiring a dynamic device is above the highest limit then a bariatric dynamic device must be selected. If the patient is below the lowest limit then a low-air-loss mattress must be selected (more information on this mattress type follows below).

Manufacturer's instructions must be adhered to, and they usually recommend that nothing other than a loose fitting sheet and /or the patient's clothing must come between the patient and the mattress/cushion as this will negate the efficacy of the dynamics (e.g. if an incontinence sheet is placed under the patient, this will be anchored on the inflated cells, which then create a bridge over the deflated cell; the incontinence sheet then presses against the patients skin, potentially causing pressure damage. This therefore brings into question the need for other devices, such as pillows to elevate heels for example.

Low air loss devices

These devices have the same indications as alternating devices, and bariatric versions are available. They are commonly used for low weight patients who have insufficient weight to 'mould' into the dynamic cells. This type of device is also beneficial to those patients who experience motion sickness from the movement of dynamic cells, and for those who experience pain with this movement. For this reason they are often the product of choice for the terminally ill.

Other commonly used devices

There is a range of other devices available that claim to relieve pressure such as heel protectors and wedges (Figure 32.6), but care /nursing staff must not forget that these devices continue to place pressure against the patient's skin, so must not be relied upon to fully relieve pressure. Regular skin checks must be carried out to ensure their continued use remains appropriate.

33 ## Pressure ulcer classification and prevention

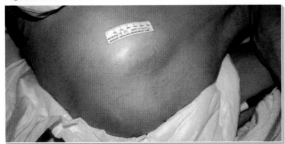

Figure 33.1   Grade I Pressure Ulcer

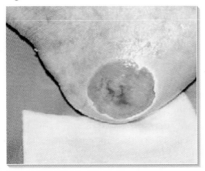

Source: Grey et al 2006, figure 5, p 473. Reproduced with permission of the BMJ.

Figure 33.2   Grade II Pressure Ulcer

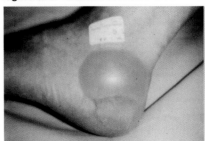

Figure 33.3   Grade III Pressure Ulcer

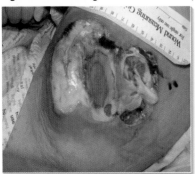

Figure 33.4   Grade IV Pressure Ulcer

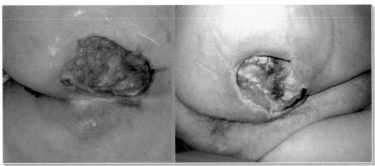

Figure 33.5   Unstageable/Unclassified (Grade III)

Figure 33.6   Deep Tissue Injury

Figure 33.7   Moisture Lesion

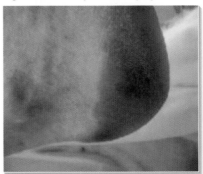
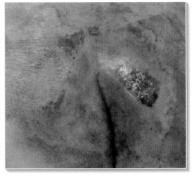

Classification of pressure ulcers

Pressure ulcers are classified in the UK using the European Pressure Ulcer Advisory Panel (EPUAP) severity scale, which uses a scale of I to IV, with Grade or Category 4 being the most severe pressure ulcer.

In the USA they use an additional two classifications that are increasingly being adopted in the UK by tissue viability nurses.

The definition of each grade/category is as follows:

Grade/Category I (Figure 33.1) – Intact skin with non-blanching redness (i.e. does not go white when pressed). This grade may be difficult to detect in darker skin tones.

Category/Stage II (Figure 33.2) – A partial thickness loss of dermis presenting as a shallow open ulcer with a red or pink wound bed. No slough or necrosis is present.

It may also present as an intact or a ruptured blister.

Category/Stage III (Figure 33.3) – Full thickness tissue loss. Subcutaneous fat may be visible but bone, tendon or muscle is not exposed.

Slough may be present but does not obscure the depth of tissue loss.

It may include undermining and/or tunnelling.

The depth will vary depending on the anatomical site of the ulcer, and is dependent on the depth of adipose (fat) tissue and muscle.

Category/Stage IV (Figure 33.4) – Full thickness tissue loss with exposed bone, tendon or muscle.

Slough, eschar (scab) or necrosis may be present.

There is often undermining and tunnelling. The depth varies by anatomical location.

USA classifications

Unstageable/Unclassified (Figure 33.5) – Full thickness tissue loss, in which actual depth of the ulcer is completely obscured by slough (yellow, tan, grey, green or brown) and/or eschar (tan, brown or black) on the wound bed.

This ulcer will be classified as a Grade III or IV in the UK.

Suspected deep tissue injury – depth unknown – (Figure 33.6) Purple or maroon localized area of discoloured intact skin or blood-filled blister due to damage of underlying soft tissue from pressure and /or shear.

The area may be preceded by tissue that is painful, firm, mushy, boggy, warmer or cooler compared to adjacent tissue. Deep tissue injury may be difficult to detect in individuals with dark skin tones.

This ulcer will be classified as a Grade III or IV in the UK.

Moisture lesions (Figure 33.7) – These are not pressure ulcers and are wounds that are caused by prolonged contact with moisture.

These are often incorrectly categorized as Grade II ulcers due to the dermal loss that occurs with maceration and/or excoriation.

This damage can however increase the speed at which a pressure ulcer will develop if not appropriately managed.

Pressure ulcer prevention

In recent years most NHS Trusts have adopted a model of care known as SSKIN, which when adopted in patient care has been proven to reduce the incidence of pressure ulcers.

It has also been proven to increase the healing rates of existing pressure damage.

However, it is important to assess and address all other influencing factors noted on pressure ulcer risk assessment as well as implementing care in accordance with the following SSKIN care bundle:

- **S – Skin** – the skin is observed on admission and any pressure damage is recorded on a Body Map.

  The Body Map is repeated each time a re-assessment of risk is carried out.

  Additionally, the patient's skin should be observed for signs of pressure damage at each position change, and at least once on every shift.

  The findings should be recorded on the care plan evaluation.

- **S – Surface** – following assessment of risk, the correct pressure relieving devices (e.g. cushions and mattresses) must be installed under the patient.

  The choice of equipment used will be determined by the holistic and risk assessment result and the specific device used must be recorded in the patient's notes (discussed in the next chapter).

- **K – Keep Moving** – NICE recommend that no patient should be left in the same position for longer than 6 hours when in bed, and no longer than 2 hours when sitting in a chair, providing the patient is on adequate pressure relieving surfaces.

  Those at greater risk will require more frequent repositioning than this, as will those who are awaiting pressure relieving surfaces.

  It is vital that every position change is recorded on a Turn/Repositioning Chart to enable continuity of care and to alert others to when repositioning is required.

  In the event that pressure damage occurs or an existing ulcer deteriorates, the frequency of repositioning must be increased without delay following re-assessment.

- **I – Incontinence** – this section must not be limited to urine and faecal incontinence, but consideration must also be given to any moisture that may be in contact with the skin for prolonged periods; for example sweat, wound exudate, or leakage from catheters or stoma bags and drink spillages.

  Adopting a regular toileting regime will prevent incontinence, whilst providing repositioning and therefore regular pressure relief for the patient.

  When there is a risk that moisture will get onto the skin it is essential that good skin care is provided using appropriate wash creams and moisture barriers.

- **N – Nutrition** – As stated in the previous chapter, reduced nutrition is the second highest reason why an individual will develop pressure ulcers.

  It is therefore vital that a nutrition assessment is completed as soon as possible after admission to the care setting, and diet and fluids are monitored to ensure adequate nutrients are taken by the patient.

  NICE recommend the use of the Malnutrition Universal Screening Tool (MUST) on admission and at weekly intervals along with weekly weights (or monthly if on a district nurse workload). Reassessments must be carried out in the event that a patient fails to take sufficient diet and fluids, or if they demonstrate any weight loss.

  In these instances food supplements must be provided and a referral to a GP or a dietician must be made without delay.

  Further, if a patient has or develops a Grade III or IV pressure ulcer, it is also advisable to refer the patient to the dietician due to the need for increased nutrition to aid healing.

34 Pressure ulcers

Figure 34.1 Pressure ulcer development

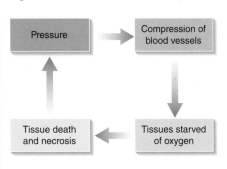

Pressure
Compression of blood vessels
Tissues starved of oxygen
Tissue death and necrosis

Figure 34.2 Common sites for pressure ulcers

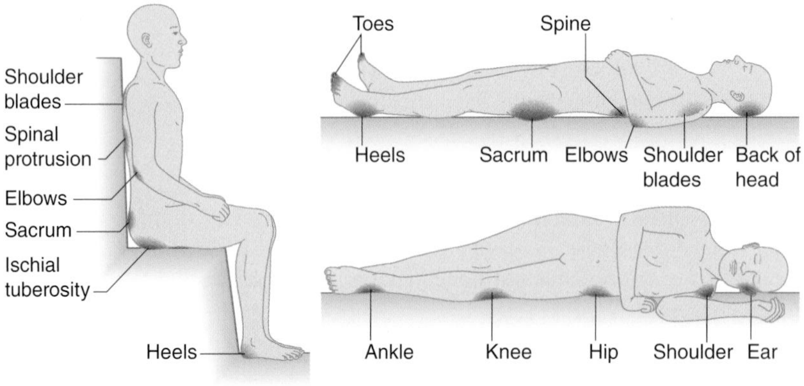

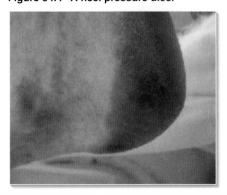

Shoulder blades
Spinal protrusion
Elbows
Sacrum
Ischial tuberosity
Heels
Toes
Spine
Heels
Sacrum
Elbows
Shoulder blades
Back of head
Ankle
Knee
Hip
Shoulder
Ear

Figure 34.3 Common sites for friction and shearing

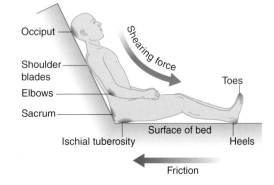

Occiput
Shoulder blades
Elbows
Sacrum
Shearing force
Toes
Surface of bed
Ischial tuberosity
Heels
Friction

Figure 34.4 A heel pressure ulcer

Wound Care at a Glance, First Edition. Ian Peate and Wyn Glencross. © 2015 John Wiley & Sons, Ltd. Published 2015 by John Wiley & Sons, Ltd.
Companion website: www.ataglanceseries.com/nursing/woundcare

Pressure ulcers are also known as bed sores, pressure sores, and pressure damage or decibitus ulcers. They can occur on any part of the body, but are seen most commonly over bony prominences such as the occiput (back of the head), sacrum, elbows, heels, hips and the ischial tuberosities (the bones we sit on) (Figures 34.2 and 34.4). One common pressure ulcer that occurs in most of us at some time is on our feet when shoes are rubbing, although most people do not recognize this as pressure damage. This chapter will deal with the causes and assessment of pressure ulcers and risk. The following chapter will deal with ulcer classification and prevention.

Aetiology

Pressure damage is predominantly caused by prolonged and unrelieved pressure from any external object against the skin (e.g. bed, chair, clothing, footwear, medical devices). The pressure applied occludes blood vessels (capillaries and venules) in the skin and underlying tissues, which means that there is insufficient or no blood supply to the affected tissues that then die due to lack of oxygen (ischaemia); further, there is a build up of waste products due to the occlusion of venules, that causes reduced tissue viability leading to poor tissue repair (Figure 34.1). It is similar to a boulder being placed on a hose pipe that feeds a garden; failure to remove the boulder to allow water through will result in the garden drying up and dying. Patients who are immobile or have difficulty responding independently to pressure, or those who have a neurological deficit and can't feel the effects of pressure, will be at immediate risk of developing pressure damage.

Additional causes

There are many factors that affect an individual's likelihood of developing pressure ulcers, and the more factors involved the greater the risk score will be, and the faster a pressure ulcer is likely to develop. It is therefore essential to carry out a risk assessment that considers all potential contributory factors so that an appropriate level of care can be planned and implemented. Here we consider some on the main factors:

Friction – is regular rubbing of the skin that removes the epithelial cells and if not protected, will damage the cuboidal cells, causing a breach to the skin, through which bacteria can enter. If pressure is applied to this area also, then a pressure ulcer will develop faster than it would otherwise do but for the friction (Figure 34.3).

Shearing – is when two tissue types are forced in opposite directions, causing tearing and inflammation at the site of trauma, usually deep within the tissues and commonly at the site of underlying bones. If pressure is applied to the area, a pressure ulcer will develop faster than it would otherwise do if shearing had not occurred (Figure 34.3).

Incontinence, moisture and sweating – moisture that is in constant or regular contact with the skin will cause maceration (i.e. water logging) or excoriation (i.e. burning) that will make the skin much more vulnerable to pressure. Skin damage from moisture will in effect give pressure damage a head start.

Poor nutrition – after immobility, reduced nutritional intake is the next main cause of pressure damage; poor nutrition leads to lethargy, reduced mobility, reduced cell regeneration, and poor healing rates. It is therefore essential the patient is encouraged to take adequate nutrition and fluids in order to reduce the risk of developing pressure ulcers and to improve healing rates in cases where they exist. The recommended daily intake for a male is around 2000 kcal and for females is around 1600 kcal per day. These calories are required for daily activities and normal cell regeneration. If a wound exists the patient will require a higher intake of nutrients, particularly of protein, in order to improve wound healing rates.

Underlying comorbidities – there are many medical conditions that make an individual more likely to develop pressure damage compared to the risk level of a healthy individual. For example, diabetes, peripheral vascular disease, other vascular diseases (e.g. vascular dementia) and coronary artery disease each have an effect on the circulation, so can affect the circulation to the skin also. When pressure is applied, the (probably) already reduced blood supply will be reduced even further, making pressure damage occur more quickly. In conditions such as malignancy, organ failure or in general malaise, the catabolic rate (i.e. tissue breakdown rate) is faster than in a health individual, which means that there is a need for increased nutrition, yet these patients usually do not feel like eating, so will be at very high risk of developing pressure damage.

Medications – certain medications are known to impact on the tissue viability of a patient; for example, steroids and cytotoxic drugs and these patients will be at increased risk of developing pressure ulcers if they are not regularly moving or repositioned.

Risk Assessment

The National Institute of Clinical Excellence (NICE 2005) recommend that all patients should be assessed for risk of pressure ulceration within 6 hours of admission to any care setting (within 24 hours on a district nurse caseload). Reassessments must be carried out a minimum of weekly (monthly on a district nurse case load), but sooner in the event the patient's condition changes, if pressure ulcers commence, or if existing pressure ulcer deteriorate. Although these timeframes are not specifically specified in the 2014 guidance, a responsible body of nurses will continue to adhere to this standard.

However, NICE warns that risk assessment tools must be used with caution and should only be used as an aide memoire only, and to evidence that an assessment has taken place. This is because for example, a patient who is completely immobile but free from any other risk factors (with a zero risk score), will be at automatic risk, whereas a patient with a very high risk score who is fully mobile and able to respond independently to pressure will be at no risk. In the event that this patient becomes immobile, then he/she will develop a pressure ulcer faster than the immobile patient with a low or zero risk score.

A word of warning: the patients that are often overlooked as being at no risk are those people living with dementia and/or learning disabilities, because they are often very mobile. However, these patients although fully mobile will be at elevated risk due to the inability of many to respond to the effects of pressure (e.g. numbness we feel when we have been sitting for too long).

35 Venous leg ulcers

Figure 35.1 Normal venous flow

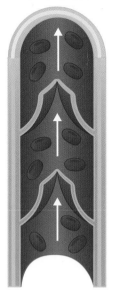

Normal vein

Source: P. Vong. Reproduced with permission of P. Vong

Figure 35.2 Incompetent venous flow

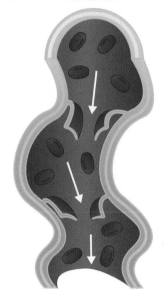

Varicose vein

Source: P. Vong. Reproduced with permission of P. Vong

Figure 35.3 Venous leg ulcer

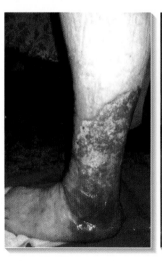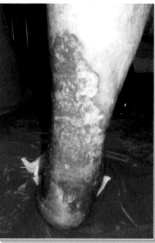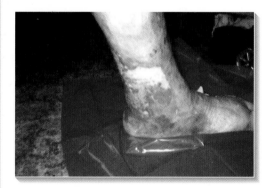

Venous insufficiency

Venous leg ulcers occur as a result of venous insufficiency and are thought to affect around 1–2% of the adult population. Venous leg ulcers are accountable for around 70–90% of all leg ulceration in the UK. Fortunately, conservative treatment will resolve most venous leg ulcers.

Aetiology

The veins are responsible for carrying deoxygenated blood back to the heart from the tissue capillaries. Venous blood contains high levels of carbon dioxide and metabolic waste collected from the tissues, which are disposed of and the blood reoxygenated as it flows through the entire circulatory system. The veins help dispose of around 90% of waste fluid, providing there is no incompetence present.

The venous system has three types of veins: deep, superficial and perforating. The deep veins lie within the muscles and are parallel to a neighbouring artery and are responsible for carrying most of the 80–90% of the blood back to the heart. Using the muscles assists with effective venous return by reducing the pressure on the vein walls from the volume of blood within, as the muscles contract it pushes the blood along the vein towards the heart, thereby reducing the venous pressures. Superficial veins lie within the more superficial tissues and are responsible for draining the skin and subcutaneous tissues. The pressures in these veins are less than in deeper veins. Perforating veins connect the deep and superficial veins throughout the lower leg.

Medium and large veins have biscuspid valves that allow one-directional blood flow (Figure 35.1). However, as blood in the legs is flowing against gravity, this places undue pressure on the valves, which can then collapse, rendering a valve incompetent (Figure 35.2). When one valve collapses this then places undue pressure on the lower valve, and so that will collapse also. As more valves collapse the entire vein, or parts of the vein will become incompetent. This incompetence then leads to venous stasis (static blood within the vein), and can lead to deep vein thrombosis, phlebitis (inflammation of the vein walls) and/or a build up of waste and carbon dioxide in the surrounding tissues. The leakage and/or build up of these waste products in the surrounding tissues can lead to spontaneous development of a leg ulcer, or in the event of trauma, a non-healing wound.

Once a vein becomes incompetent it is irreparable, so venous insufficiency will become a lifetime condition. On occasions a vascular surgeon may remove a vein in order to minimize the risk of thrombosis; however, this then places increased pressure on surrounding veins as the venous return re-routes itself, which increases the risk of further venous incompetence.

Risk factors

Inactivity of the calf muscle is the main cause of venous incompetence and leg ulceration, e.g. sitting or standing still for long periods. Other factors are previous venous ulceration, advancing age, trauma, pregnancy, smoking and diabetes mellitus.

Symptoms

The symptoms of venous insufficiency can include mild to moderate pain that is relieved on limb elevation; oedema; cellulitis (skin infection); brown staining (pigmentation); induration (i.e. lumpy texture of underlying tissues due to the build up of lymph and waste products); itching, and skin is less elastic than healthy tissues. Where a wound exists, healing rates will be poor, if at all (in undiagnosed ulcers); the ulcer is usually located on the gaiter area of the leg just above the bi-malleolus, the ulcer is usually shallow with sloping edges, and can be extensive in aspect that may cover the circumferential aspect of the gaiter area; there is usually a large amount of wound exudate due to the escape of oedema resulting from the venous incompetence (Figure 35.3). In the absence of arterial disease (discussed later) foot pulses are usually present and the feet are usually warm to touch and pink in colour.

Diagnosis

As always, diagnosis is made following holistic and clinical assessment. The clinical assessment will include a Doppler ultrasound assessment in order to obtain an ankle–brachial pressure index (ABPI), which will confirm or rule out any arterial involvement. This is important as the treatment for venous insufficiency is usually contraindicated in the presence of arterial insufficiency (discussed in other chapters). A normal ABPI is between 1.0 and 1.2

Treatment of venous insufficiency

Intervention is aimed at reducing the venous hypertension and providing mechanical support by way of compression hosiery or bandaging to the incompetent veins. Activity that uses the calf muscles must be encouraged and prolonged sitting or standing must be avoided. Elevation of the legs so that they are slightly higher than the heart should be encouraged as this will ease pressure off the valves and allow gravity to remove the waste products instead. Venous insufficiency means a lifestyle change must be adopted as it is an incurable condition that means the patient will always be at risk of leg ulceration and non-healing traumatic wounds.

Treatment of venous ulcers

Good skin care is essential so on removal of the compression therapy, wash the patients leg with emollients (using a basin with tap water is adequate), pat the peri-wound skin and leg dry with a clean soft towel and apply emollients to the skin, avoiding the wound itself and between toes. Apply the most appropriate dressing following assessment of the wound (see chapters on wound treatments and dressing choices), and reapply the compression therapy. It is common for compression bandages to be used when an ulcer exists due to the difficulties in applying compression hosiery. Once the ulcer heals compression hosiery can be used on a continuing basis in order to avoid recurrence of the ulcers.

36 Lymphoedema

Figure 36.1 Cavity wound on a lymphoedematous limb treated with larval therapy

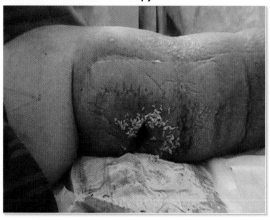

Figure 36.2 Lymphoedema of the left leg. The right has chronic oedema

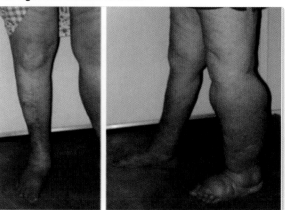

Source: Lawenda et al., 2009, p. 14. Reproduced with permission of John Wiley & Sons.

Figure 36.3 Lymphoedema of the upper limb following mastectomy and removal of axillary lymph nodes

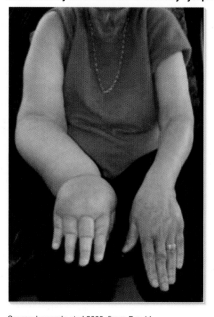

Source: Lawenda et al 2009, figure 7, p. 14.
Reproduced with permission of John Wiley & Sons, Ltd.

Figure 36.4 Unilateral lymphoedema with a healthy right leg

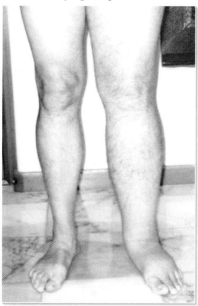

Source: Lawenda et al., 2009, Figure 6, p. 13.
Reproduced with permission of John Wiley & Sons.

Wound Care at a Glance, First Edition. Ian Peate and Wyn Glencross. © 2015 John Wiley & Sons, Ltd. Published 2015 by John Wiley & Sons, Ltd.
Companion website: www.ataglanceseries.com/nursing/woundcare

The lymphatic system

Lymphoedema is a condition in which there is an accumulation of protein-rich lymph fluid due to a deformation or destruction of lymph nodes or there is impaired transport of lymph around the body. It can affect any part of the body depending on what part of the system or lymph nodes affected by congenital defect, trauma, surgical removal or disease. Typical onset of primary lymphoedema is at birth and at puberty in males and females; and at first pregnancy and the menopause in females. Secondary lymphoedema onset results from disease (e.g. cancer), trauma and chronic oedema.

The lymphatic system has two main functions: it assists with the regulation of fluid in the body, ridding the body of around 10% of waste fluid per day, absorbing larger molecules than the venous system can deal with. Therefore, together the venous and the lymphatic system will remove 100% waste fluids from the body each day; also, it is part of the immune system.

The lymphatic system is part of the circulatory system and in effect it is recycling blood plasma around the body. This fluid, known as lymph, travels through a network of vessels similar to the venous and arterial systems; it flows into progressively larger vessels and is pushed along by skeletal muscle contraction and the respiratory pump towards larger 'collectors' and on to regional lymph nodes. If any part of this system is destroyed or impaired for any reason, the fluid will not reach its destination and will accumulate in the tissues below the affected vessels, collectors, or lymph nodes. Lymph nodes contain lymphoid cells that produce lymphocytes, which assist the body's immune system.

Regional lymph nodes are located in areas such as the ankle, knee and groin, which remove lymph fluid from the lower limbs into the lower abdomen nodes, and in the wrist, elbow, neck and axilla, which remove lymph from the head and upper limbs into the chest and then the upper abdomen nodes.

When any of these nodes are damaged or diseased, the lymph fluid accumulates in the tissues up to the affected lymph node, causing an increase in size of the affected limb (Figures 36.1–36.4). Elevation of the limb does not allow drainage of this excess fluid, and current treatments are restricted to massage and compression bandaging that force the lymph from the tissues and back towards the lymphatic system for drainage.

Skin care

It is essential that good skin care is encouraged using wash creams and emollients (discussed in Chapter 30), ensuring that the skin and skin folds are fully dried prior to the application of these products. As the limb increases in size, the skin folds require exceptional care to avoid fungal infections, soreness from maceration/sweating and pressure damage from the weight of skin on skin.

Compression

The application of compression therapy must only be applied when diagnosis and treatment has been confirmed. It must only be applied by a practitioner who has been trained and is competent in the practice of lymphoedema compression bandaging. The pressures used in lymphoedema compression therapy are usually higher than for venous ulceration; in the UK this is usually at around 50 mmHg pressure.

Prior to the application of compression, careful preparation must be afforded to applying wadding to the folds in order to protect from pressure and to ensure the limb is structured into a cylinder shape. The compression is then applied from the tip of each individual toe, along the foot and up to the groin. As the lymph fluid is squeezed into the major lymph node in the groin for disposal, the limb is gradually reduced in size. The bandages then need to be removed and immediately reapplied to further reduce the lymph and size of the limb. This process must be followed until such time that the limb is reduced to an acceptable size, and compression must be continually applied thereafter in order to prevent a build-up of lymph in the limb again.

When the upper limb is affected, care must be taken to ensure rings are not tight; it is advisable to remove rings as the size of the limb will inevitably increase without treatment, and could therefore compromise the arterial supply to the fingers.

Wound management

The primary treatment is to deal with the underlying cause of the lymphoedema and this should entail a referral to a specialist centre so that an accurate diagnosis can be made before treatment is commenced. Failure to manage this condition will delay wound healing.

In the meantime, it is important to carry out a holistic assessment in order to identify any influencing factors that could contribute to additional delays in wound healing.

When a wound occurs on a limb affected by lymphoedema there will be an elevated risk of cellulitis and/or wound infection due to the lack of lymph drainage and reduced immunity due to ineffective lymphatics. It is therefore vital that wounds are avoided as far as possible by the provision of good skin care and by avoiding using the affected limb for venepuncture or cannulation as far as possible.

In most cases, the principles of wound healing and treatments will apply as discussed in other chapters.

Conclusion

Limbs affected by lymphoedema will require referral to and a treatment plan by a specialist. In the meantime, it is essential that good skin care is provided, tight-fitting garments and rings removed, and only trained and competent clinicians apply compression therapy to affected limbs. Following holistic assessment, wounds must be treated in accordance with the principles of wound management detailed in other chapters.

Compression therapy

Figure 37.1 3M Coban 2 compression system bandage

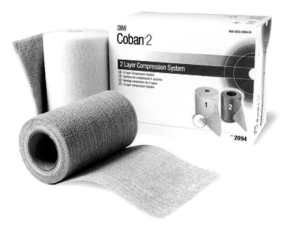

Source: Image © 3M. Reproduced with permission of 3M.

Figure 37.2 Compression hosiery

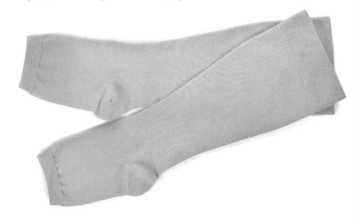

Source: iStock © Geo-grafika.

Box. 37.1 Laplace's Law

$$\text{Bandage compression} = \frac{\text{Tension/layers applied/constant}}{\text{Limb girth/bandage width}}$$

Table 37.1 Layers of compression and the pressure each provides

ABPI	Layers used	mmHg
>0.8	All four layers	35–40
0.7	Layers 1, 2 and 4	23
0.6	Layers 1, 2 and 3	17
<0.5	Compression contraindicated	0

Table 37.2 Layers of compression and the pressure each provides

Class 1	14–17 mmHg
Class 2	18–24 mmHg
Class 3	24–35 mmHg

Compression therapy is used to treat venous insufficiency, with or without the presence of venous ulceration. Venous insufficiency is a result of venous hypertension brought about by incompetent non-return valves located on the inside walls of the vein. If treatment is not provided for this condition the tissue integrity surrounding the affected veins will be reduced, and in some cases ulceration will occur.

What is meant by compression?

Compression therapy is the application of a compressive force around the affected limb by way of compression bandages (Figure 37.1) or compression hosiery (Figure 37.2). This therapy enhances the functioning of the venous valves, thereby reducing venous hypertension, aiding venous return. This improves the tissue integrity as waste products and toxins are expressed from the tissues back into the veins for disposal via the correct route (e.g. the kidneys).

There are two types of compression bandage systems: multilayer bandages and short-stretch bandages. The system selected must be applied in accordance with the manufacturer's recommendations and by a health professional trained and competent in the application of this therapy. Compression hosiery is an alternative method of compression; however, it is very difficult to apply to a limb because of the lack of elasticity so is rarely used when an ulcer is present.

Ultimately, all compression systems are aimed at supporting the structure of vein walls that have become varicosed because of their incompetence. Compression can only be applied where there is no evidence of arterial insufficiency; otherwise the circulation to the limb, particularly the skin, will be reduced by the compression. Therefore, it is essential that the health professional is aware of when compression is contraindicated (refer to flow chart in Chapter 40).

In the UK, the optimum therapeutic level of compression is around 40 mmHg at the ankle, reducing to around 17 mmHg below the knee.

Laplace's Law

The amount of pressure applied to a limb is referred to as Laplace's Law; the amount of compression applied can be increased by applying a narrow bandage or by increasing the number of layers applied. If the stretch on the bandage (as recommended by the manufacturer) is maintained at the same level the pressure will decrease as the bandage is wound around the limb, thereby having the greatest pressure at the ankle, which then reduces as it rises to below the knee. Box 37.1 shows how the pressures are calculated according to Laplace's Law.

Multilayer systems

These consist of up to four layers, the top two layers forming the compression layers. By omitting one of the top two layers there is a reduced level of compression applied. Reduced compression is used in cases where mild peripheral vascular disease may be present, but reduced compression should only be used under specialist supervision. Multilayer systems are suitable for the immobile patient or for those who have an ineffective calf muscle pump, as the pressures remain constant even when immobile. The layers are as follows:

1 The first layer consists of absorbent wadding. It protects bone prominences from pressure damage and is used to shape the limb into an inverted 'cone' shape in order to distribute pressure. More padding is used on smaller circumference ankles of less than 18 cm and no greater than 25 cm, in order to achieve no more than 40 mmHg pressure around the ankle.
2 The second layer is a crepe bandage which secures the wadding and serves as an additional absorbent layer.
3 The third layer consists of an elastic bandage that provides 17 mmHg at the ankle.
4 The fourth layer is a cohesive bandage that provides 23 mmHg pressure at the ankle.

Therefore the third and fourth layers combined provide 40 mmHg compression, and this provides full compression commonly used when there is an ABPI of >8. When reduced compression is required this will be determined by the ABPI result (Table 37.1).

When ankle circumference is greater than 25 cm this reduces the sub-bandage pressure an additional cohesive compression layer will be required, although this would be applied in the opposite direction to the original layer.

Short stretch systems

These systems require the patient to be mobile with an effective calf muscle pump in order to achieve full compression when walking. At rest the compression will be significantly reduced, so is often more tolerable to patients. These bandages are usually two layer systems, with wadding being the first layer in order to shape and pad the limb. The second compression layer is applied at full stretch in order to create a firm cylindrical pressure around the limb, which when the patient walks the muscle is forced against the 'cylinder' causing the blood in deeper veins to be compressed, forcing the blood back to the heart.

Compression hosiery

Hosiery is usually used as a maintenance treatment for venous insufficiency to prevent ulcer recurrence, and is usually applied once an ulcer has fully healed. Standard sizes and made to measure are available with different classes of compression (Table 37.2). Patients wearing hosiery or bandages must only do so under medical advice and must have their ABPI monitored on a regular (e.g. 3-monthly) basis.

38 Arterial ulcers

Figure 38.1   Arterial ulcer

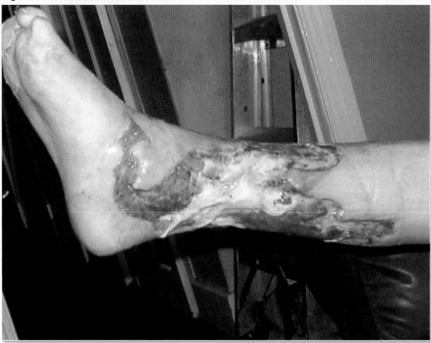

Figure 38.2   Arteriosclerosis

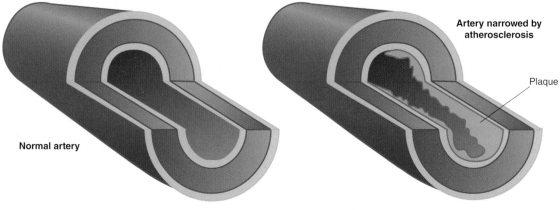

Normal artery

**Artery narrowed by
atherosclerosis**

Plaque

Source: P. Vong. Reproduced with permission of P. Vong.

Wound Care at a Glance, First Edition. Ian Peate and Wyn Glencross. © 2015 John Wiley & Sons, Ltd. Published 2015 by John Wiley & Sons, Ltd.
Companion website: www.ataglanceseries.com/nursing/woundcare

Arterial insufficiency

Arterial insufficiency, often called peripheral arterial disease (PAD) is the lack of, or a reduction in, the blood supply. It is found in varying degrees of severity amongst sufferers ranging from mild PAD to critical ischaemia (i.e. tissue death due to no blood supply). PAD of the lower extremities accounts for around 10% of all leg ulceration in the UK. However, a leg ulcer could be of venous, arterial or mixed (i.e. both arterial and venous) aetiology and it is important to identify what type of ulcer you are dealing with, as the treatments required for each are very different. It is vital that priority consideration is given to the presence of PAD when treatments are being considered. The causes, diagnosis and treatment of venous ulcers are dealt with in previous chapters. In this chapter we will look at the causes, diagnosis and treatments of arterial ulceration (Figure 38.1).

Aetiology and risk factors

Blood circulates from the heart to every cell in the body via the arterial system, first via larger arteries (e.g. aorta) then branching into smaller main arteries, then into smaller arteries and then into capillaries, which are found at the tip of the arterial tree. Arterial blood delivers oxygen and nutrients to cells to maintain health and life, without which tissues will die.

There are many reasons why arterial insufficiency occurs, including arteriosclerosis (plaque development in the lumen of the artery/capillary, Figure 38.2); destruction of capillaries from disease (e.g. diabetes), from smoking and from high blood pressure (hypertension); trauma, and/or unrelieved pressure, and from age-related changes that cause vasoconsolidation (hardening of the arteries) or vasoconstriction (narrowing).

Medical conditions such as coronary heart disease, diabetes, stroke, vascular diseases such as vascular dementia or organ failure due to vascular disease make it more probable the patient will also develop PAD. Additionally, any patient with PAD will be at increased risk of developing pressure ulcers (discussed earlier).

In PAD it is common for the tip of the arterial tree to be affected first, so the skin and the extremities and their underlying tissues will be at risk of tissue death. This can result in reduced tissue integrity in the mildest of cases, to onset of or the non-healing of existing wounds. In the severest conditions, it can result in gangrene of the limb (e.g. commonly in the toes/feet in diabetics) due to the complete occlusion of one or more arteries. The tissues that will be affected will depend on which artery (or arteries), or capillaries are blocked.

Symptoms

It is most common that symptoms will have an insidious onset to begin with whereby no symptoms are obvious. However, there are occasions when a sudden blockage of an artery will occur that will cause excruciating ischaemic pain for the individual. For patients with the former type of PAD, the symptoms gradually increase over time and can include one or more of the following classic signs:

- thin, shiny, hairless legs (or patches of hair loss)
- thickened toenails (reduced blood supply to the nail bed)
- pale, cool feet (pales and cools further on limb elevation)
- foot discolouration (can be very red, or black)
- poor tissue perfusion (i.e. capillary refill >4 seconds). Capillary refill time reduces on limb elevation
- weak, or absent foot pulses (sounds heard on Doppler may fade on limb elevation)
- limb pain which worsens on limb elevation and which is relieved by lowering the limb
- pain on walking, relieved by resting (intermittent claudication)
- severe pain on resting
- non-healing leg wounds, that have a deep, punched out appearance with steep edges.

Diagnosis

As always, diagnosis is made following holistic and clinical assessment of the limb. A Doppler ABPI assessment can be carried out to confirm the nurse's suspicions of vascular disease; however this may not be tolerated well by the patient due to the pain likely to be experienced. In the event that an ABPI is obtained that is outside of the normal range of 1.0–1.2, the patient should be referred to a vascular team for further assessment and a duplex scan in order to determine the extent of the PAD and to determine the most appropriate treatment. Where a normal range ABPI is obtained, but the patient experiences any of the above symptoms, PAD must be considered as a possibility. In the meantime, where PAD is suspected based on assessment findings, care must be taken to avoid any compression therapy, tight clothing or footwear until the patient has been assessed by the vascular team.

Treatment

Treatment options will vary depending on the findings and severity of the PAD. In many cases an angioplasty can be performed to stretch/sweep the narrowed artery to increase blood flow. This often produces temporary improvements and repeat angioplasties are necessary. Occasionally, where larger arteries are blocked or narrowed, surgery can be performed in order to remove the blockage or to reroute the arteries by way of bypass grafts. However, in cases where it is the capillaries that are blocked or damaged no treatment is available, and it is a case of treating the patient holistically by providing education on lifestyle choices and education on skin care.

Where a wound is in existence it is essential that best practice in wound care is provided so that the wound can heal as quickly as possible, at rates that will be determined by the level of blood supply to the wound bed. In many cases a wound will fail to heal regardless of the wound treatments applied because there is an insufficient blood supply to the wound bed.

39 Doppler

Figure 39.1   Doppler. NBVV = non-bleeding visible vessel

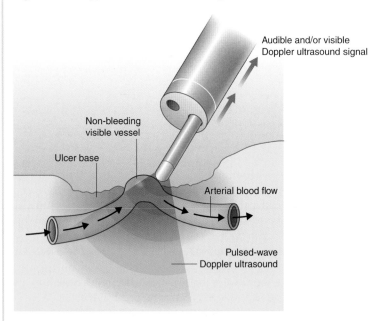

Audible and/or visible
Doppler ultrasound signal

Non-bleeding
visible vessel

Ulcer base

Arterial blood flow

Pulsed-wave
Doppler ultrasound

Figure 39.3   Some Dopplers also produce a visual wave form reading

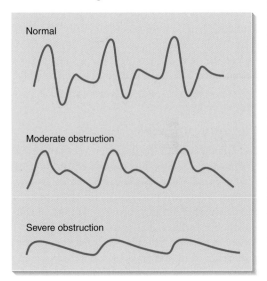

Normal

Moderate obstruction

Severe obstruction

Figure 39.2   Doppler equipment and application

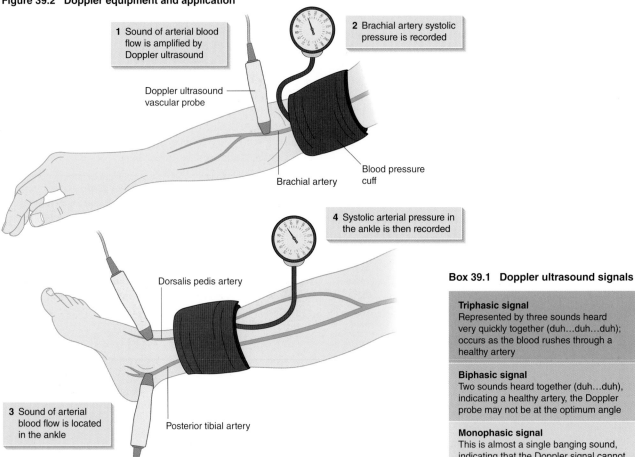

1 Sound of arterial blood
flow is amplified by
Doppler ultrasound

2 Brachial artery systolic
pressure is recorded

Doppler ultrasound
vascular probe

Blood pressure
cuff

Brachial artery

4 Systolic arterial pressure in
the ankle is then recorded

Dorsalis pedis artery

3 Sound of arterial
blood flow is located
in the ankle

Posterior tibial artery

Box 39.1   Doppler ultrasound signals

Triphasic signal
Represented by three sounds heard
very quickly together (duh...duh...duh);
occurs as the blood rushes through a
healthy artery

Biphasic signal
Two sounds heard together (duh...duh),
indicating a healthy artery, the Doppler
probe may not be at the optimum angle

Monophasic signal
This is almost a single banging sound,
indicating that the Doppler signal cannot
penetrate a diseased artery. This sound
is usually lower in pitch

Predicting non-healing wounds is not always clear-cut. A reliable diagnosis requires information about both the macro- and the microcirculation. Ultrasound, angiography and peripheral pressure indexes such as ankle/toe–brachial index are often used to assess the microcirculation. Microcirculation can be diagnosed using laser Doppler technology. Using a Doppler effectively requires a skilled practitioner.

Doppler

Generally, all stages of peripheral arterial disease should be verified and confirmed using objective tests such as the ankle–brachial index (ABI) and Doppler. Laser Doppler technology is a non-invasive method and is an investigative tool. A laser light is used to detect blood perfusion in the microcirculation (Figure 39.1). The measuring depth is approximately 0.5–1 mm, reaching the superficial vessels:

- arterioles
- venules
- shunts
- capillaries.

Doppler relates to the change in frequency of a wave as the source or target moves. When used as part of a vascular assessment, the technique uses the direction and velocity of blood flow to determine whether the patient's arterial blood vessels are healthy or diseased. It is the brachial and ankle systolic pressures that are measured using a hand-held Doppler probe at the brachial pulse and the dorsalis pedis pulse on the dorsum of the foot. The ankle pressure is divided by the brachial pressure to obtain the ankle–brachial pressure index (ABPI).

Doppler assessment can be used in a variety of situations, commonly used when assessing a person with a leg ulcer; this chapter concentrates on leg ulcer assessment. Doppler ultrasound is performed by listening to signals transmitted from the Doppler probe.

Performing Doppler

The practitioner must provide information that the patient can understand and that is relevant to their circumstances enabling them to make an informed decision; information should include details of the possible benefits and risks. Treatment should take into account any factors, such as physical or learning disabilities, sight or hearing problems, or difficulties with reading or speaking English and appropriate adjustments made.

Patient preparation

The patient will be asked to lie as flat as possible, with one pillow for the head and the procedure will take between 10 and 20 minutes, assuming this position removes the effect of gravity on blood flow. If the patient is unable to assume this position, they should be asked to lie as low as is possible. The patient may experience some discomfort as the blood pressure cuff is placed on the ankle and as it is inflated. If at any time the patient finds the procedure too painful, they can ask for it to stop it at any time. The patient should remove any tight items of clothing, which may cause pressure on the blood vessels proximal to the site where the blood pressure is being measured. Remove any dressings from the ulcers and cover with vapour-permeable film dressing or equivalent to reduce risk of cross-infection.

Equipment required

The following equipment will be required (see Figure 39.2):

- a Doppler ultrasound with an 8-Mhz probe
- a sphygmomanometer and the appropriate size blood pressure cuff for the shape and size of the patient's arms and ankles
- sterile cover to the ulcer bed (prevents cuff irritating the ulcer bed, helps to promote comfort and prevents contamination of the cuff), vapour-permeable film dressing or equivalent
- ultrasound gel, used as a contact medium between the patient and the Doppler probe
- chart for recording pressures.

The procedure

Two practitioners should work together to perform the procedure, one of whom should be a trained in Doppler use and assessment. The patient should be asked to lie flat for 10 minutes prior to the procedure beginning (unless contraindicated); this will help to avoid the unwanted effect of gravity.

Apply the blood pressure cuff to the upper arm. Locate the brachial artery through palpation and apply transducer gel to that area. Hold the Doppler probe at 45 degrees over the area of skin that has the gel on it and move the probe until the clearest signal has been located. Inflate the blood pressure cuff until the signal disappears, slowly deflate the cuff and listen for the signal to re-emerge; record. Carry out the same test on the other arm and record the highest pressure as the brachial systolic pressure, which will be compared against the ankle pressures.

Expose the ulcer and cover in a vapour-permeable film dressing or equivalent. Locate the pedal arteries. There are four of these:

1 anterior tibial artery
2 posterior tibial artery
3 peroneal artery
4 dorsalis pedis artery.

Two of the four are used, the most common are the most accessible: the dorsalis pedis and the posterior tibial arteries. Apply the blood pressure cuff above the malleoli; apply transducer gel over the artery. The Doppler is applied over the artery and the best signal detected. The blood pressure cuff is slowly inflated. Listen for the Doppler signal to disappear as the pressure exerted in the cuff occludes the artery. Slowly deflate the cuff; observe and note the pressure at which the Doppler signal reappears; record this pressure for that artery. Enquire how the patient is. Locate one of the other pedal arteries and repeat the process. If the blood pressure cuff cannot compress the artery, this indicates severe disease (see Figure 39.3 and Box 39.1).

After obtaining all of the readings, make the patient comfortable and slowly assist them to the upright position. Inform the patient what you have done and what will happen next. The practitioner must perform Doppler ultrasound in addition to obtaining a detailed health history and this will incorporate the patient's social circumstances.

All findings should be recorded.

40 Interpreting ABPIs

Figure 40.1   Flowchart for the management of ABPIs

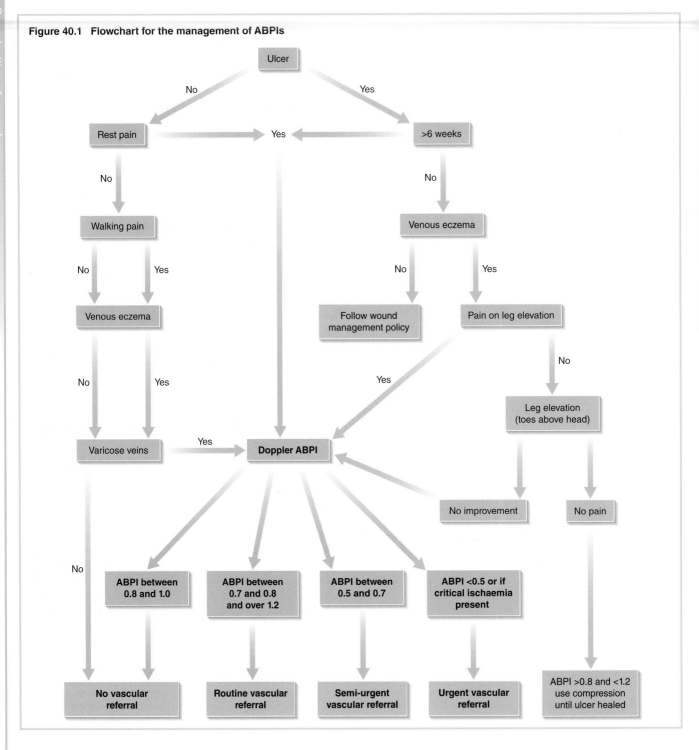

Wound Care at a Glance, First Edition. Ian Peate and Wyn Glencross. © 2015 John Wiley & Sons, Ltd. Published 2015 by John Wiley & Sons, Ltd.
Companion website: www.ataglanceseries.com/nursing/woundcare

An ABPI result must not be considered in isolation when it comes to management of leg ulcers; it does however confirm or rule out any vascular disease, which will indicate when not to apply compression therapy. When performing a Doppler assessment, it is equally if not more important to examine the entire limb for signs of underlying conditions that may indicate vascular or venous disease. It is also important to ask the patient about pain and any aggravating factors that may exacerbate pain.

The flow chart in Figure 40.1 will prompt the questions and symptoms to look for and which must be considered when carrying out an ABPI and holistic assessment. The chart will also guide the nurse on the most appropriate management for the patient.

When performing a Doppler assessment, it is important to first locate the foot pulses and listen to the sounds of the blood flow as this can determine how healthy the arteries actually are and whether or not the ulcer is likely to be of artery or venous origin. Secondly, the ABPI result will determine whether or not compression therapy is appropriate or whether a referral to a vascular surgeon is appropriate and whether or not that referral should be dealt with on an urgent basis or not. The flow chart in Figure 40.1 will assist with the decision-making process; however, local policies and guidelines must be adhered to.

Artery sounds

1 *Triphasic sounds* – will be audible by Doppler ultrasound as the vessel expands and relaxes in rhythm with the heart beating and blood circulation. A triphasic beat indicates a healthy artery.
2 *Biphasic sound* – as blood reaches the lower extremities (i.e. the feet) the sound fades in most adults and only two beats may be heard. A biphasic beat indicates a healthy artery.
3 *Monophasic sound* – if only one beat is heard (usually a loud whooshing sound) this indicates a calcified (hardened) vessel. The walls are less elastic than a healthy artery, often due to age or disease such as diabetes. The sound is often much louder than with a healthy artery as the blood flow causes echoing within the artery.

Monophasic sounding arteries

The monophasic beat is an indication that the blood vessel is unhealthy, and it is most probable that the vessel will be difficult to compress when performing an ABPI due to the calcified state of the artery wall. If the vessel is incompressible by 180 mmHg pressure, then the ABPI on that vessel must be abandoned as any result above this will be false.

When a vessel is compressed the cut-off and re-entry sound pressures must be noted; the sound of a healthy artery will cut off and re-enter at the same mmHg pressure, whereas a calcified vessel will have a slower sound re-entry than the point at which the vessel was completely occluded. This is because a healthy artery is more flexible and will occlude easier with direct pressure than a calcified artery, which will be harder to occlude and slower to spring open thereby causing the delay in the sound re-entry.

ABPI results and referral pathway

A normal ABPI is regarded as between 1.0 and 1.2. Providing there are no other clinical signs of vascular disease, compression therapy is usually recommended.

ABPI above 1.2 or if compression above 180 mmHg pressure is required to occlude the artery sound is usually indicative of calcified vessels, and compression ought to be avoided until the patient has been assessed by a vascular surgeon.

An ABPI between 0.8 and 1.0 does not usually require any intervention and providing there are no other clinical signs of arterial compromise it is usually acceptable to apply compression therapy; however, close monitoring of the ABPI and clinical inspection of the limb must be undertaken on a regular basis (e.g. monthly) to observe for deterioration in the vascular status of the limb.

ABPIs between 0.5 and 0.8 indicate that there is a flow of arterial blood to the feet, the degree of which is indicated by the ABPI. The urgency of the referral will depend on the result (refer to the flow chart). There may be associated pain on limb elevation or on walking (claudication).

When the ABPI is <0.5 and/or if foot pulses are absent, it will be common for the patient to complain of severe resting pain, which collectively may be indicative of critical ischaemia and will require an urgent referral for further investigation and opinion.

Calculating ABPIs

When calculating ABPIs, it is common practice that the highest brachial pulse is used to calculate the ABPI against all pulses. Similarly, it is the highest foot pulse that is used to calculate the ABPI on each foot. However, care must be taken not to overlook the lowest foot pulse on each foot as this could indicate that that particular vessel is partially occluded and using the highest foot pulse could mask a problem in the neighbouring artery.

Undertaking an ABPI requires training and competence by the nurse undertaking the procedure as an incorrect calculation or procedure could lead to inappropriate or contraindicated care being provided. Incorrect treatment could lead to increased pain, delayed healing or compromised circulation in the event that compression therapy is applied when it ought to be contraindicated.

41 Diabetic foot ulcers

Figure 41.1   Diabetic leg and foot ulcers

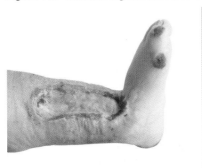

Source: Shutterstock © Svitlana Kazachek

Figure 41.2   Pressure ulcer on the diabetic foot

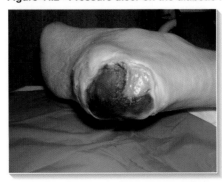

Figure 41.3   Sloughy neuropathic foot ulcer

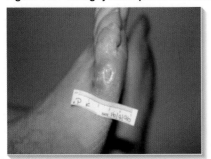

Figure 41.4   Neuropathic foot ulcer after maggot therapy

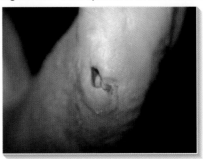

Figure 41.5 (a,b) Diabetic foot ulcers with gangrenous (black) areas

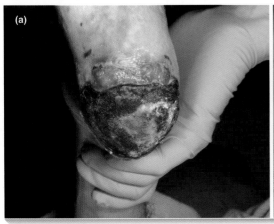

(a)

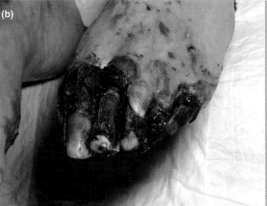

(b)

Wound Care at a Glance, First Edition. Ian Peate and Wyn Glencross. © 2015 John Wiley & Sons, Ltd. Published 2015 by John Wiley & Sons, Ltd.
Companion website: www.ataglanceseries.com/nursing/woundcare

Diabetes is a condition where the pancreas fails to produce sufficient insulin, or at all, and sugar levels in the blood increase as a result. This in turn causes destruction of blood vessels, thereby causing many conditions as a consequence. For example, patients with diabetes have an increased risk of conditions such as dementia, vascular disease, multi-organ failure, glaucoma and loss of sight, and in terms of tissue viability, foot and leg ulcers (Figure 41.1) that could potentially lead to amputation.

Diabetes has two types (Type I and Type II); the risk of the latter increases with age and obesity, and is becoming an increasing phenomenon in the developed world with more people developing Type II diabetes than ever before.

The diabetic patient can develop a foot wound spontaneously or in the event that a wound occurs for other reasons (e.g. surgery, trauma and pressure) they are notoriously difficult to heal. Furthermore, the risk of infection is increased in the diabetic due to the reduction in blood supply (and therefore white blood cells) to the wound bed.

The diabetic patient often develops neuropathy, which makes it unlikely the patient will feel the pain of any trauma that occurs. This often means that diabetic foot wounds are overlooked until such time that they become saturated with exudate and/or become infected and a malodour is noted by the patient. Prevention is therefore much better than cure.

Foot surveillance, foot checks and foot care

First and foremost, it is crucial that a diabetic patient undergoes regular (annual) foot checks with a diabetic podiatrist so that the structure, sensation and vascular status can be monitored in accordance with NICE (2011). The patient or care staff should thereafter monitor the patient's feet for signs of callus (hard skin) that may have underlying ulcers, for any signs of trauma (e.g. from footwear) and for the onset of any wounds that may occur spontaneously. In any such event, it is crucial to provide excellence in wound management and to ensure a prompt referral to a diabetic foot specialist is made without any delay.

It is crucial that correct fitting footwear is used and the diabetic podiatrist will be best placed to give advice on this.

Foot complications

The diabetic patient will have an increased risk of developing pressure ulcers due to their compromised circulation and the possible presence of neuropathy, which means they are unable to respond to the effects of pressure, so will remain in the same position, thereby compromising the circulation further, causing necrosis (tissue death) as can be seen in Figures 41.2–41.4.

As a diabetic patient's foot structure changes, they can develop a condition called Charcot osteoarthropathy, which causes the instep to collapse as the bone structures collapse, often causing the appearance of flat feet or a 'rocker' sole, which then makes the patient more vulnerable to pressure damage; thus observation of the foot and prompt referral is vital to prevent wounds occurring.

Wound management

Generally the principles of wound management apply in the diabetic foot ulcer as with any other wound; however, due to the increased risk of wound infection and often the presence of tissue death (gangrene) there are some very important points that require discussion:

Gangrene – this is dead tissue caused by a lack of or no blood supply and is often a feature of a diabetic foot ulcer (Figures 41.5). The lack of oxygen causes ischaemia and subsequent tissue death, which has a black (necrotic) appearance. The tissues will die until it reaches a healthy blood supply, after which the gangrene usually auto-amputates providing it is allowed to remain dry (or is dried out), and the wound will then heal at that point. It can affect one part of the foot (e.g. one toe), or the entire foot (also involving the leg) and may in critical cases require surgical amputation in the event of increased pain or the risk of gas gangrene.

Gas gangrene – this is dead tissue that is affected by a gas-producing bacterium known as *Clostridium perfingens*. The gas produced by the bacteria liquefies and then breaks down tissues, which can then rapidly place the patient's limb or life at risk. This particular bacterium thrives in moist to wet environments and is unable to survive in dry environments. Indeed, this bacterium is present in most soils on earth except in deserts, and it is this bacterium that is responsible for decomposing dead bodies. Bodies have been preserved in desert sands for thousands of years because this bacterium does not exist in deserts. Therefore, in the event that an ischaemic limb where gangrene exists (including any other necrotic tissues), care must be taken to dry out the affected tissues in order to prevent the rapid production of this bacteria and the potential to destroy a limb or cause the patient's death by sepsis often within 24–48 hours.

Moist wound healing – this is contraindicated in the gangrenous wound and is only recommended when there is a wound bed that is free from gangrene (or any other necrotic tissue e.g. black slough/debris) and when the blood supply to the wound bed is very good. If the blood supply is good to the wound bed so the immunity will be good (via the white blood cells), so will afford the diabetic patient some protection from infection.

In the event that necrosis or gangrene is moist, then the tissues must be covered with an absorbent dressing (e.g. a foam) in order to dry the wound out. In the meantime, a sustained release antimicrobial dressing ought to be applied directly to the gangrenous/necrotic tissues in order to reduce the bacterial bio-burden on the wound bed in order to minimize the risk of infection, and most importantly, of gas gangrene.

When there is no gangrene (wet or dry) or any necrotic debris present, then it is reasonable to apply the principles of wound healing in the management of the diabetic foot ulcer.

42 Moisture lesions

Figure 42.1 Moisture lesion on the buttocks

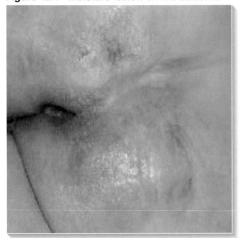

Figure 42.2 Blanching erythema

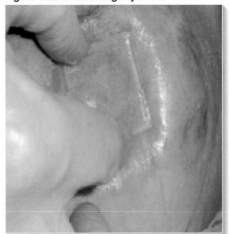

Figure 42.3 Non-blanching erythema
Grades 1, 2 and 3 pressure damage

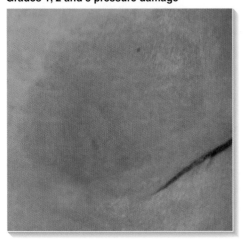

Figure 42.4 Grade 4 pressure damage

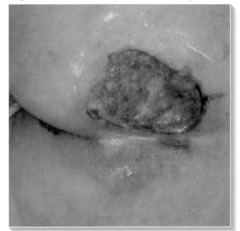

Table 42.1 Differences between moisture lesions and pressure ulcers

Pressure ulcer	Moisture lesion
Usually occurs over a bony prominence such as over the sacrum, or under anything that applies constant pressure to the skin, e.g. under the tight elastic on underwear	Occurs where there is excess moisture against the skin. The area may be extensive and over areas where there are no bones immediately underneath the skin, e.g. the buttocks, groins
Usually round in shape to begin with and confined to the area directly over the bone	Appears initially as a rash or a tiny graze(s) that is sporadic over the area of moisture
The onset of pressure damage appears red (when it is a Grade 1). When pressed it is non-blanching (i.e. it remains red when pressed, Figure 42.3)	Appears red, and when pressed the red area blanches (i.e. it goes white)
The skin surrounding the ulcer is usually dry	The skin around the lesions appears 'wet'
The depth of damage can go deep down to muscle, bones and tendons	Is usually superficial, although if pressure is applied on these areas, the damage can go deep as with pressure ulcers. These ulcers will be categorised as pressure ulcers, with a moisture lesion onset
Can become infected, although this is unusual with good wound management. Therefore any infection will be delayed, if at all	Can usually become infected very quickly due to the presence of bodily fluids and matter that harbours bacterial growth
Usually hot or lumpy to touch	Usually cool to touch, unless infected
The patient complains of pain	The patient usually complains of a stinging sensation

Moisture lesions are areas of the skin that are damaged by excessive and prolonged contact with moisture such as sweat, incontinence of faeces and urine, from wound exudate or from spillages (Figure 42.1). Initially the skin becomes wet and the dead skin cells absorb the moisture. This then causes the skin to become macerated (i.e. soggy or water-logged). Eventually the maceration reaches the cuboidal cells rendering them penetrable by bacteria and so the skin is breached and an open wound occurs. The resulting skin damage is usually very superficial and usually destroys the epidermal and the dermal layers of the skin (Figures 42.2 and 42.3). The extent of the damage will depend on the extent that the moisture spreads, and so can often result in widespread destruction (Figure 42.4). This type of wound occurs commonly under skin folds such as under the breasts, under the abdominal apron, and around the buttocks, groin, sacrum and vulval areas. As a result, fungal infections commonly occur on these lesions, giving a very red and excoriated (burning) appearance. Moisture damage in effect will give pressure damage a head start, so it is vital that adequate pressure relief is provided. Moisture lesions are often mistaken for pressure ulcers but Table 42.1 details the subtle differences between the two types of skin trauma.

A moisture lesion or a pressure ulcer?

The differences between moisture lesions and pressure ulcers are given in Table 42.1.

Prevention and management of moisture lesions

As always, prevention is much better than cure; therefore, to begin with, as far as possible, it is vital to address the cause of the incontinence (or sweating, or both). This may include instigating a regular toileting regime (e.g. two or three times hourly) and excellence in skin care in the event that incontinence occurs. In any event it is essential that expert advice is sought from a Continence Specialist Nurse, who will be able to assess, treat and manage the cause of your incontinence.

In the meantime, as well as the above, it is crucial that the following care is taken in order to avoid moisture lesions:

1 The application of appropriate sized continence pads; these must be fitted to the conformity of the body and should not be placed as a sheet under the patient. Modern pads have an indicator when they need changing (e.g. a line that appears on the outer pad). Choosing the right sized pad will mean that maximum wear time and costs will be achieved; the pad will be changed before it reaches its maximum absorbency, after which the moisture will then sit against the skin. It is therefore important to look for the indicator line. However, this method of capturing moisture must not be a substitute for toilet opportunities.

2 The use of an appropriate moisture barrier cream that will assist in preventing moisture sitting next to the skin. It is important to be aware of the variety of products on the market, thereby following expert advice. Many barrier products are difficult to spread onto the skin due to the consistency; applying and washing off the barrier cream can cause skin trauma. Furthermore, some barrier creams (e.g. Sudocrem) are contraindicated for use with continence pads, as this product (as well as others) can 'clog' the pores of the pad, thereby preventing moisture soaking into the pad. This results in moisture sitting against the skin, which will eventually penetrate the cream, causing moisture damage. It is therefore advisable to use tissue viability recommended barrier creams such as Cavilon cream.

3 Once there are breaks in the skin caused by moisture (and/or pressure ulcers), it is advisable to stop the use of creams and use a barrier spray instead (e.g. Cavilon spray). This creates a 'protective film' that moisture is unable to penetrate. Applying creams to moisture lesions will simply add to the moisture levels, which will encourage further bacterial growth, thereby increasing the risk of cellulitis.

4 Keep skin clean and dry, using a moisturizing barrier cream (e.g. Cavilon cream) as already stated. Avoid the use of alcohol wipes and soaps to wash the skin; use wash creams instead (e.g. Tena wash cream). Soaps containing alcohol causes the skin to dry and crack, so when urine or faecal matter get on to the skin this will cause a stinging sensation and increase the risk of infection.

5 Ensure adequate nutrition and hydration. A good well-balanced diet and around 2 litres of fluids daily will maintain maximum skin integrity.

6 If the patient is unable to reposition themselves independently in response to pressure, it is vital that care is provided to ensure regular repositioning is carried out in order to prevent pressure ulcers occurring; as moisture lesions will give pressure damage a 'head start' and they can quickly deteriorate to deeper tissue damage.

43 Surgical wounds

Figure 43.1   A surgical adhesive strips

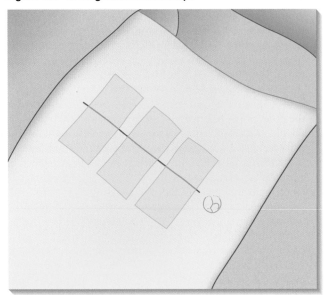

Figure 43.2   Paper strip dressing

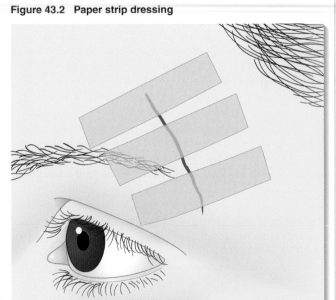

Figure 43.3 Staples

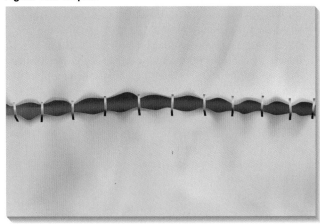

Figure 43.4 Sutures

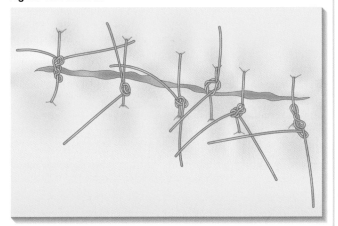

Source: P. Vong. Reproduced with permission of P. Vong.

Wound Care at a Glance, First Edition. Ian Peate and Wyn Glencross. © 2015 John Wiley & Sons, Ltd. Published 2015 by John Wiley & Sons, Ltd.
Companion website: www.ataglanceseries.com/nursing/woundcare

Most surgical wounds are closed at the time of surgery with the wound edges held together with mechanical aides such as sutures, staples (clips), paper strips or glue, or a combination of these aides. This type of closure is known as primary intention. As a result the wound will have a minimal exposed surface area with very little tissue loss, and in most cases the wound will heal fully within 3–4 weeks as it follows the healing process, which has been described in earlier chapters. However, on occasions the wound will dehisce (i.e. burst open) for a variety of reasons and will require healing by secondary intention, which means that it will require appropriate dressings to create an optimum environment to encourage it through the healing process.

Postoperative wound care

Postoperative complications include bleeding and wound infection. In the event of bleeding, it is vital that this is arrested by using firm pressure, applying alginates that contain haemostatic properties (e.g. Kaltostat) directly to the wound, and if not arrested within 20 minutes it is vital that the patient is referred to a medical officer without delay.

At least 5% of patients undergoing a surgical procedure will develop a surgical site infection that may become evident within 7–10 days post operation (CG74, NICE 2008). Postoperatively an interactive (insulating) dressing must be applied to the surgical wound. In most cases the dressing is best left undisturbed for the first 48 hours, after which it should be removed to observe for signs of infection and dehiscence. If the dressing becomes saturated with wound exudate, if bleeding is observed, if there is a sudden increase in pain or if a malodour is noted, then the dressing should be removed for observation and wound assessment. Dressing replacement should be applied by use of the 'aseptic non-touch technique'.

Wound irrigation

If the wound requires irrigating (i.e. usually when there is any loose debris or excess exudate), sterile saline should be used during the first 48 hours postoperatively. After this time tap water is considered safe for use on wounds. The wound is usually considered 'waterproof' after 48 hours, so it is usually acceptable for patients to take a shower after this time, although they should avoid using wash products on the wound.

Wound dehiscence

There are several reasons why a wound will dehisce; swelling caused by the trauma of the surgical procedure; obesity; too much tissue loss causing greater tension on the wound closure; and infection or underlying abscess formation. Each of these will put too much tension on the mechanical aids used to close the wound, thereby causing the wound to dehisce. Many cases of dehiscence are unavoidable, but with good wound management these wounds will usually heal well by secondary intention.

However, wounds that heal this way tend to have larger scars, which will be weaker in tensile strength than the previous tissues and will have a poorer cosmetic result than a scar that has healed by primary intention.

Documenting a surgical wound

Although it is anticipated that most surgical wounds will heal spontaneously and will require little intervention, it is essential that the wound site, size and wound closure aids are documented as a minimum to begin with. On first review or dressing change (whichever is sooner) of the wound the nurse should record the condition of the surrounding skin and suture line as a baseline condition. In the event of dehiscence the wound ought to be fully assessed and the findings documented on a Wound Assessment Chart (see Figure 20.1).

Removal of sutures, staples, paper strips and adhesive

Adhesive (Figure 43.1) It is not necessary to remove adhesives from wounds and should be left to auto-debride from the wound.
Paper Strips (Figure 43.2) Must be kept dry until they are due for removal at around 7 days. It is advisable to soak the strips before removal; lift the strip from both outer edges towards the suture line, then gently remove them from the wound. If a wound dehisces, it is not necessary to reapply strips to hold the edges together and secondary intention healing should be applied.
Staples (Figure 43.3) It is not necessary to cleanse the wound before or after staple removal. Staples are usually removed in 7–10 days unless specified otherwise. Special disposable staple removers are used to remove these aids.
Sutures (Figure 43.4) It is not necessary to cleanse the wound. There are two types of sutures; removable and dissolvable.

• Removable sutures are usually black or navy blue in colour and are usually removed at 7–10 days post operation, unless specified otherwise. The sutures can be one long subcutaneous stitch or can be individual sutures. It is important for the nurse to determine the number and type of sutures used before removal in order to ensure the correct care can be provided.
• Dissolvable sutures are usually flesh (pale pink) or violet coloured. This type of suture does not require removal and will dissolve when in contact with subcutaneous exudate in around 60–71 days.

Once mechanical aids have been removed it is essential that the wound continues to be observed for any signs of dehiscence, infection, and over time of abnormal scar tissue formation, each of which will require referral to a medical office for appropriate intervention.

44 Traumatic wounds

Figure 44.1 Incision/cut

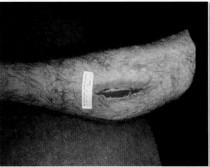

Figure 44.2 Laceration

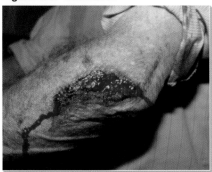

Figure 44.3 Puncture wound

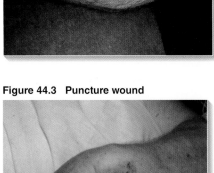

Figure 44.4 Abrasion/friction

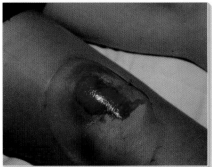

Figure 44.5 Contusion/bruise

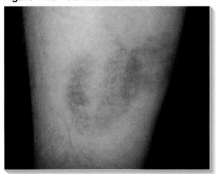

Wound Care at a Glance, First Tradition. Ian Peate and Wyn Glencross. © 2015 John Wiley & Sons, Ltd. Published 2015 by John Wiley & Sons, Ltd.
Companion website: www.ataglanceseries.com/nursing/woundcare

Traumatic wounds are caused by a sudden or unplanned external insult. There are many types of traumatic wounds, which may include injuries from road traffic accidents, gunshot wounds, domestic accidents, trips and fall and burns from heat, cold, electricity and chemicals.

The principles of wound healing should be applied in all cases; however, many traumatic wounds will require thorough irrigation and/or debridement both initially and ongoing through the wound healing process, as required. It is essential that the wound is protected from further trauma, and the choice of dressing can go some way to achieve this. As with any wound, the underlying cause of the wound must be identified and either eliminated or controlled in order to avoid recurrence of the injury; for example, if an individual is spilling a hot drink on their on a regular basis, action must be taken to avoid such spillages (e.g. reducing the heat of the drink). The following descriptions are of common wound types caused by trauma. A brief outline of each follows.

Incision (cut) (Figure 44.1) – usually caused by a 'slice' to the skin and underlying tissue by a sharp-edged implement, a shard of glass, scalpel, knife, sheet of metal. The edges are usually clearly defined with little, if any, tissue loss. The edges of the wound can be held together without undue tension by mechanical aides (e.g. clips, sutures, strips, adhesive or a combination of these). As these wounds will heal by primary intention, they require minimal wound care after closure. A hyrdofibre and a film dressing would be an appropriate dressing, which will promote healing as this will allow absorption of exudate, which will usually be minimal in these wound types.

Laceration (Figure 44.2) – usually caused by a blow from a blunt object, causing the skin to split/tear into a skin flap, particularly over a bony prominence. A common example of this type of wound is the pre-tibial laceration. The skin flap can be thick or thin depending on the extent of the tissue destruction. There is often some skin/tissue loss noted, and often the edges do not meet due to surrounding swelling caused by the injury. Where little or no swelling occurs the wound can often be healed by primary intention. If there is any tissue loss or extensive swelling the wound must heal by secondary intention. Often a combination of wound closure is required. In either type of closure, it is vital that this wound is thoroughly irrigated to get rid of loose debris, and the flap edges should be rolled back in order to allow epithelial to epithelial tissue repair. The mechanism of injury will indicate if the tissues are likely to swell which will assist with the decision-making process regarding choice of wound closure. A hyrdofibre and a film dressing would be an appropriate dressing, which will promote healing, as this will allow absorption of exudate, which will usually be minimal in these wound types.

Skin tear – this injury is usually caused by the skin being torn on a sharp object, such as a nail, or a fingernail. It is often regarded as a laceration, and wound closure will be determined by the amount of tissue loss, if any as with lacerations. It is vital that the wound is thoroughly irrigated before closure to evacuate debris from the wound in order to reduce the risk of infection. A hyrdofibre and a film dressing would be an appropriate dressing, which will promote healing, as this will allow absorption of exudate, which will usually be minimal in these wound types.

Puncture/penetrating (Figure 44.3) – these wounds are caused by a sharp, pointed implement penetrating into deep tissues or by a bone fracture piercing through the skin and underlying tissues (as seen in Figure 44.3), a bullet wound, or a bite (animal, human or insect). On removal of the cause the puncture wound may appear small and insignificant, but should not be underestimated; damage to underlying structures is highly probable with this type of wound (e.g. tendon, internal organs, nerves, blood vessels) as is the risk of infection. It is vital that these wounds are thoroughly explored by a medical officer and/or X-rayed to ensure there is no remaining foreign body or underlying trauma before the wound entry site is closed. Often antibiotics are given in high-risk injuries such as bites (particularly punctures caused by a cat bite).

Burn/scald – can be caused by heat, cold, electricity or chemicals (see Chapter 47); it is vital that the cause of the burn is identified before treating:

- *Heat* – wounds ought to be cooled by using cold running water, or ice wrapped in a towel
- *Cold* – burns (often called frost bite) must not be warmed up but protected with a clean towel to prevent further heat loss
- *Electricity* – first and foremost the rescuer must ensure their own safety and switch of the electric supply before attending the patient. The patient needs to be admitted to the emergency department to check for cardiac function as electricity can cause internal burns and affect heart rhythms.

Abrasion/friction (Figure 44.4) – this is a wound that results in superficial dermal loss, but friction can cause deep abrasions depending on the mechanism of injury and indeed can result in full thickness tissue loss. The skin is generally subject to low levels of friction on a daily basis, which may cause thinning of the dead epithelial layers initially, but could traumatise the protective cuboidal cells (the living layer of the epidermis) resulting in an open wound. Common areas that are affected with friction are the heels and elbow. In areas at risk a film dressing can be applied, which will offer protection to vulnerable areas; and in the event of trauma hyrdofibre and a film dressing would be an appropriate dressing, which will promote healing as this will allow absorption of exudate, which will usually be minimal in these wound types.

Contusion/bruising (Figure 44.5) – this occurs due to trauma against tissues causing a rupture to a blood vessel(s) that allows blood to seep out into the surrounding tissues causing a haematoma. It is important to arrest the bleeding to reduce the size of the haematoma. Initially the bleed will produce a 'red' and often swollen appearance to the skin and as the underlying wound ages the deoxygenated blood will darken, causing discolouration commonly called a 'bruise'. It is therefore regarded as a 'closed wound'. A contusion may be present around other wound types caused at the time of the injury, and commonly presents with a laceration due to the extensive effect of the blunt trauma affecting wider tissues. If there is no breach to the skin around the contusion, then no specific dressing is required, and the venous return and lymphatic drainage will eventually disperse the haematoma, which will resolve usually within 10–14 days.

45 Burns and scalds

Figure 45.1 Chemical burn (cement)

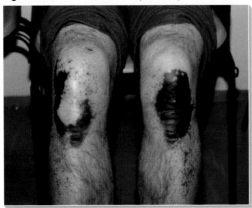

Figure 45.3 Sunburn

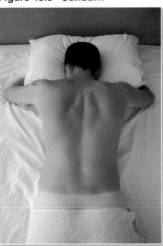

Figure 45.2 Body Map showing the rule of nines

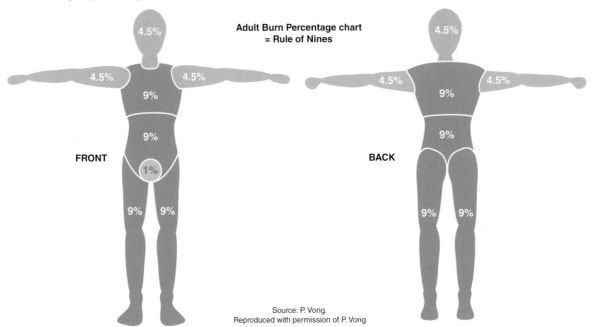

Adult Burn Percentage chart
= Rule of Nines

FRONT

4.5%
4.5%   4.5%
9%
9%
1%
9%   9%

BACK

4.5%
4.5%   4.5%
9%
9%
9%   9%

Source: P. Vong.
Reproduced with permission of P. Vong

Table 45.1   Estimated total body surface area calculated using the rule of nines

Anatomical area	% TBSA
Head/neck	9
Each arm	9
Anterior thorax	18
Posterior thorax	18
Each leg	18
Perineum	1

Table 45.2   Features of varying depths of burns

Superficial partial thickness of the epidermis	Red but without blistering. Not usually life threatening; no scarring
Superficial dermal	May have small blistering and/or total epidermal loss. The area is usually wet due to loss of interstitial fluid. Usually has minimal scarring. Blanches (goes white) when pressed
Deep dermal	Total epidermal loss or blistering, red in appearance, does not blanch when pressed and there is loss of sensation. Scarring is likely

The origin of tissue destruction by burns and scalds must be identified as each type of trauma requires different management strategies. Scalds are caused by hot liquids or steam and burns are caused by hot or cold objects, fire, chemicals (Figure 45.1) or electricity. The first aid of each trauma type can be found in Chapter 46, so this chapter will focus on the long-term management of each type of burn/scald.

Assessment and resuscitation

First and foremost, it is vital that an assessment of the burns and total surface area affected is established out and resuscitation applied as necessary, depending on the total body surface area (TBSA) affected. Burn severity greater than 20% TBSA will require intravenous fluid infusion; burns greater than 30% TBSA could prove fatal. In children these percentages are much less and any burn/scald affecting even just 5% will require hospitalization. Table 45.1 represents an estimated TBSA in adults using the *rule of nines* (Figure 45.2), a commonly used method in the UK to estimate the extent of burns.

Severity

The severity of a burn is determined by the surface area and the depth of the affected injury. The depth of different types of burns is described in Table 45.2.

Burns or scalds that are circumferential or affecting moveable areas such as the palm of hands, over joints and on the face will require medical attention irrespective of size, as the maturative phase of wound healing can lead to contractures, thereby limiting movement and/or causing deformities. The greatest risk to patients with burns is infection due to the skin's breach over a large area; therefore, aseptic technique when dealing with burns/scalds is paramount. Silver antimicrobial dressings are commonly used on burns (e.g. Aquacel Ag) in order to provide the patient with a protective barrier.

Management of burns

Minor burns (Figure 45.3) – first aid includes reducing the heat by running under cold water. Wrap the burn in 'cling-film', covered by a towel, and apply ice to continue the heat reduction. Ongoing wound management should include removal of the loose skin, leaving blisters intact to minimize the risk of infection. Non-adhesive dressing should be applied (e.g. Aquacel) directly to the affected area and covered with an occlusive absorbent dressing (e.g. Mepilex). The wound should be reviewed after 24 hours. Pain relief can be provided. In the event of infection, daily dressings and antibiotics will be required.

Major burns – first aid may include upper airway management, so immediate medical help must be called for. Preventing further fluid loss by wrapping the burns in cling-film; keeping the patient warm to reduce their risk of hypothermia as they will have lost their ability to control body temperature due to excess skin loss. DO NOT apply cold water or ice to the burns as this will cause hypothermia. These patients should be referred immediately to a specialist burns unit as soon as they have been medically resuscitated and stabilized.

Chemical burns (Figure 45.1) – irrigate the chemical for long periods in large amounts of water, sometimes this can be for as long as 10 hours in cases of alkali burns (e.g. cement). Using a urine dipstick against the wet skin over the burn can identify when irrigation has been sufficient (when a normal 5.5 pH has been achieved). Irrigation may be necessary for longer periods, particularly if the eye has been affected.

Referral to a specialist burns unit

In many cases the patient will require the specialist medical attention of a specialist burns unit and it is vital that the patient with any of the following is transferred to the unit without delay immediately they have been medically resuscitated and stabilised for transfer. The following list is not exhaustive and any patient with a wound that you are uncertain of must be referred to a burns unit for specialist advice:

- any child under the age of 5 or an adult over the age of 60 years who has sustained a severe burn must be transferred to a specialist unit without delay
- patients with circumferential burns
- those with burns to their face, hands, over joint or on the perineum
- chemical burns affecting 5% of the body surface area
- any patient with exposure to chemicals or radiation
- any patient with any underlying medical conditions/comorbidities
- pregnant women
- large affected areas (5% for the under 16 age group) and 10% of the over 16 age groups.

46 Atypical wounds

Figure 46.1 Bullous pemphigoid

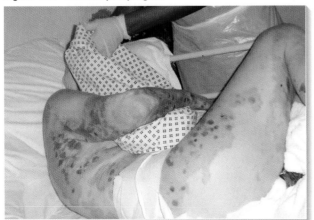

Figure 46.2 Cutaneous TB under the tongue

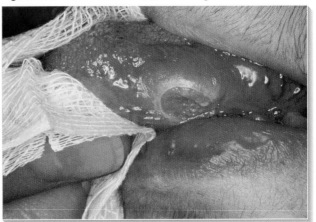

Source: CDC Public Health Image Library.

Wound Care at a Glance, First Edition. Ian Peate and Wyn Glencross. © 2015 John Wiley & Sons, Ltd. Published 2015 by John Wiley & Sons, Ltd.
Companion website: www.ataglanceseries.com/nursing/woundcare

Atypical wounds

Atypical wounds are those that are of unknown origin or those that present in unusual sites and with abnormal presentation. It is thought that many of these wound types are caused by conditions such as malignancy and rare illnesses. They tend to fall into the causation categories of inflammatory wounds, autoimmune disease, infective wounds, external cause or genetic/hereditary causes. This chapter will consider the most common types of atypical wounds that the average nurse is likely to encounter in his/her nursing career.

Bullous pemphigoid (Figure 46.1) – this is a rare autoimmune condition that generally affects the elderly population. It occurs when the immune system forms antibodies that then attack its own tissues. Blisters occur that can become painful and as this is an autoimmune disease renders the patient at increased risk of infection via these skin breaches along the dermis/epidermis junction. On occasions these blisters present in the mouth and throat and the intestinal tract; they can also occur in the trachea, and this is a life-threatening situation that requires immediate hospital admission for mechanical ventilation. The mainstay treatment for this condition is steroids. The wound treatment priorities are to protect the patient from infection as far as possible by using antimicrobial dressings that also provide a moist environment in order to prevent adherence and pain.

Pyoderma gangrenosum – this is a rare condition that causes skin ulceration and inflammation for unknown reasons. It can often be found in traumatic wounds, particularly in those patients who may unknowingly have this condition. The lesions usually occur as red, elevated eruptions that resemble insect bites and can be very painful. Wound treatments are as with any other wound type, but may include the application of topical steroids, following advice of a specialist dermatologist.

Blastomycosis – this is a rare infection cause by inhaling fungi from soil, wood or plants. It can cause skin lesions and is associated with breathing difficulties and by bone and joint pain.

Cutaneous tuberculosis (Figure 46.2) – this is caused by the invasion of the same bacteria that causes pulmonary tuberculosis. The skin lesions present as purple or re/brownish watery growths and commonly affect the limbs and buttocks. The lesions may persist for years and can clear up without any active treatment, however some lead to limb amputations. Treatment is usually with antibiotics and topical antimicrobial treatments that may be required for several months or years.

Scleroderma – this is a chronic autoimmune condition that presents as inflammation and tissue fibrosis (skin hardening and tightening), discolouration and itching. It can be very painful, especially as the skin hardens.

There are many other less common atypical wounds; however, in most cases the principles of wound healing apply in order to promote healing, prevent or eliminate infection and to prevent trauma. Therefore the use of non-adherent antimicrobial dressings and specialist advice on the treatments of the underlying causes

(once diagnosed) must be adhered to. If in doubt, refer the patient to a member of the dermatology or tissue viability team.

One very common atypical wound condition that most nurses find difficult to deal with is that of hypergranulation. It is therefore important to discuss this in this section, although it could be regarded as a normal, although unwanted, aspect of wound healing.

Hypergranulation (over-granulation) – a wound of any type can appear to progress towards healing very nicely until such time that it begins to over-granulate; then the progression to healing appears to stop. Occasionally, it will proceed without intervention but often it will not progress until the wound environment is altered from moist to dry. Hypergranulation commonly occurs around drain sites (e.g. suprapubic catheters and PEG sites) and can be problematic for the nurse and painful for the patient. The cause of hypergranulation is important to understand so that it can be avoided and/or treated in a timely fashion.

- *Appearance* – hypergranulation appears like healthy but raised/swollen granulation tissue that often sits proud to the surrounding skin level. The term hypergranulation suggests that there are more granulation cells growing than would usually be expected; however, this is incorrect.
- *The cause* – this situation is thought to result from high levels of bacteria, the waste products of which alter the pH levels on the wound bed, that then traumatizes the granulation cells, preventing them from maturing and 'shrinking' to their normal size. Their appearance is larger than would otherwise be but for this phenomenon. Once this situation occurs it is difficult for the wound to progress to healing until the condition of the wound is altered to reduce bacterial levels, which in turn will regulate the pH levels on the wound bed; any granulation cells that are produced will continue to remain swollen, and epithelial cells are reluctant to migrate across the altered pH levels of the wound until it is rectified.

Treatment and prevention – in order to rectify the wound conditions and to allow maturation of the granulation cells and the migration of epithelial cells there are two options available: (i) absorbing all of the moisture from the wound to dry out the wound bed using a foam dressing; this changes the environment the bacteria have become familiar with and so they will die. Once the wound is dry the granulation cells will mature and shrink, then moist wound healing can be reintroduced so that healing can be promoted; and (ii) the application of an antimicrobial dressing (ideally one that will not achieve a moist environment (e.g. Actisorb silver or Acticoat) which will kill the bacteria that causes the problem, covered by a foam dressing to absorb moisture. Once the situation is rectified and a dry environment is achieved, the hypergranulation tissue will reduce in size and healing will progress as normal, so moist wound healing can resume. In the event that exudate levels rise the nurse must be alert to the recurrence of this situation as bacterial levels increase once again, so repeat interventions will be required until resolved once again.

Figure 47.1 'Homelessness: it makes you sick' campaign poster

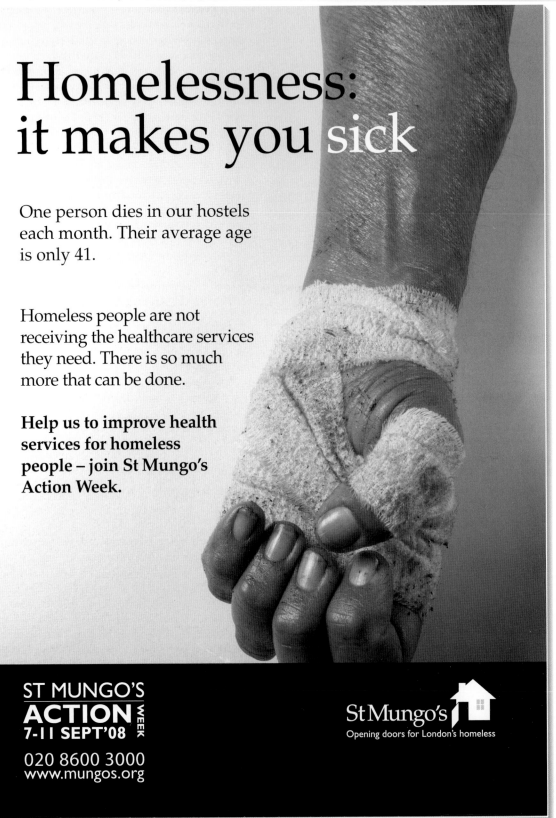

Homelessness:
it makes you sick

One person dies in our hostels each month. Their average age is only 41.

Homeless people are not receiving the healthcare services they need. There is so much more that can be done.

Help us to improve health services for homeless people – join St Mungo's Action Week.

ST MUNGO'S
ACTION WEEK
7-11 SEPT'08
020 8600 3000
www.mungos.org

St Mungo's
Opening doors for London's homeless

Source: St Mungo's Broadway, 2008. Reproduced with permission of St Mungo's Broadway.

Wound Care at a Glance, First Edition. Ian Peate and Wyn Glencross. © 2015 John Wiley & Sons, Ltd. Published 2015 by John Wiley & Sons, Ltd.
Companion website: www.ataglanceseries.com/nursing/woundcare

Hard to reach, seldom heard

There are some members of our community who are 'hard to reach' through traditional healthcare services; they are sometimes referred to as:

- seldom heard
- socially excluded
- easy to ignore
- hidden populations.

Commissioners and providers of wound care services and other statutory and voluntary organizations working with hard-to-reach groups can achieve better outcomes through targeted action to identify at-risk patients early and providing intensive clinical and social support to help them.

Traditional hospital and primary care services are not always the best way of reaching and treating some groups of people and services can be hard to access for some vulnerable people. People who are hardest to reach include:

- those with drug or alcohol addiction
- asylum seekers and refugees
- homeless and insecurely housed people
- gypsies and travellers
- those within the criminal justice system
- people with learning disabilities
- people with long-term mental health problems.

Older people and those with mental health illness or learning disabilities have worse health experiences than the rest of the population. Access to primary and secondary care differs among populations, as does the quality of some of these services; this, in turn, impacts on health outcomes.

The homeless, drug users, migrants and those in prison are not homogeneous groups; it is acknowledged that many of them are difficult to contact. There are certain groups who are particularly 'hard to reach' and highly mobile. Society tends to marginalize, isolate and socially exclude some groups. They are often not in contact with any statutory, and in some instances voluntary services, they may be unaware of them or they chose not to access them.

They may find it difficult to recognize problems with their wounds and to access diagnostic and treatment services. They may also have problems in self-care and attending regular appointments for clinical follow-up. This can lead to incomplete treatment with serious consequences.

Homeless and insecurely housed people

Accessing healthcare is often problematic for homeless people, due to difficulties in registering with a GP, problematic appointment systems, lack of access to a phone or transport, disordered lifestyles and some may have experienced discriminatory attitudes by healthcare providers.

People who are homeless have rates of physical ill health that are many times greater than those of the general population. Addressing and treating their health needs can be challenging, sometimes due to missed appointments, comorbidities, lack of concordance and poor nutrition.

Factors that increase homeless people's risk for acute and chronic wounds include communal living and eating, lack of facilities for washing and toileting, unsafe and unsanitary shelters, exposure to crime and trauma, inadequate nutrition, no place for bed rest, no place to keep medications, excessive smoking and drinking, little or no income and absence of family and other support to help in times of illness. Substance abuse and mental illnesses may affect a person's ability to understand and follow a wound care treatment plan.

These factors are associated with the homeless person, the service and the practitioner:

- concordance and 'buy in' from the patient, attendance at clinic, assessment, diagnosis and treatment
- a non-judgmental approach and good relationships
- clinic accessibility
- prescribing and accessibility of specialist wound care products, that meet the needs of the person's life style
- effective multidisciplinary working with the community
- consideration and treatment of co morbidities
- provision or referral to other services.

The therapeutic relationship

The value of a good rapport with patients is sometimes underestimated. Most service providers are clearly health focused. There is also a need for value service delivery in a framework of general social support, advocacy, assisting and non-judgmental care.

Relationships with service providers are often valued more than treatment options or therapies provided, it is important to attend to this basic human need first. The therapeutic relationship is one that offers the other respect, trust and care.

A relationship that conveys acceptance and support to patients may reduce levels of cortisol that is often elevated when a person is anxious or has concerns about health. Raised cortisol levels have an impact on wound healing, practitioners should adopt actions to minimize stress and in so doing the healing response is likely to improve.

Homeless people die earlier than the rest of the population, homelessness is associated with higher mortality.

Services can adopt an outreach approach, this is an effective strategy in reaching and targeting 'hard to reach' populations providing a service that is accessible and flexible in approach. While outreach is important and valuable, it is just as important to ensure that centre-based services are designed in such a way that they can accommodate the 'hard-to reach'. Those providing wound services should commit themselves to establishing imaginative and innovative responses to meet the needs of this vulnerable group.

Fair access to primary and secondary care for some people in the UK remains problematic. The experiences of people from hard-to-reach groups offer important insights into barriers to accessing care. There is a need to provide local care that is pluralistic, adaptive and holistic; in order to ensure that there is equitable access to wound care services.

Appropriate dressing choice and skilled wound management are certainly essential aspects of wound healing; there are a number of other physical and psychosocial factors that are equally important. At the heart of effective health care provision is a successful therapeutic relationship between practitioners and patients.

48 Malignant wounds

Figure 48.1   Fungating malignant breast wound

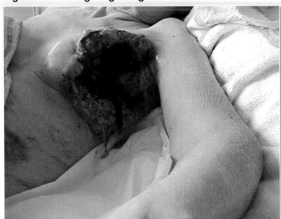

Figure 48.2   Fungating leg ulcer

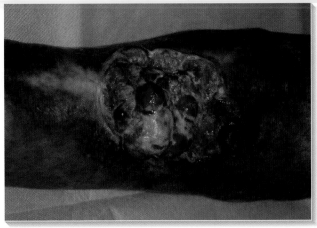

Source: Onesti et al 2013, figure 4a, p. 3. Reproduced with permission of John Wiley & Sons, Ltd.

Figure 48.3   Early-stage malignant wound, often mistaken for hypergranulation tissue

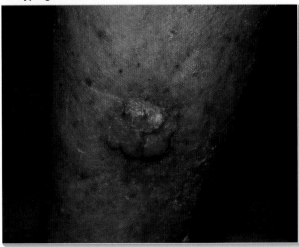

Source: Onesti et al 2013, figure 2, p. 2. Reproduced with permission of John Wiley & Sons, Ltd.

Wound Care at a Glance, First Edition. Ian Peate and Wyn Glencross. © 2015 John Wiley & Sons, Ltd. Published 2015 by John Wiley & Sons, Ltd.
Companion website: www.ataglanceseries.com/nursing/woundcare

Malignant wounds are also known as malignant tumours, fungating ulcers, cancerous wounds or ulcerating wounds. The description of a fungating ulcer is derived from the appearance of the wound that grows in the shape of a fungus or a cauliflower (Figures 48.1 and 48.2). Most malignant wounds develop in cancers that affect the breast, head, neck, skin and groin or anal areas, but can also occur anywhere on the body. Unless the cancer is eradicated, these wounds fail to heal and so the aims of care is to maintain an optimum control of the symptoms these wounds can produce, such as malodour, high levels of exudate and increased levels of pain, while protecting the surrounding skin from additional damage from poor wound care techniques and choices.

Why malignant wounds occur

Malignant wounds occur when underlying disease (cancer) causes a wound to erupt through the skin. Sometimes the malignancy starts in the epithelial cells of the body to form a wound. The malignancy may be of a primary origin (where the cancer originates) or can be spread from other parts of the body to form a new, secondary cancer on another part of the body, and may or may not produce a wound. In any event a medical diagnosis is required to determine whether or not any wound on a cancer patient is related to the malignancy.

In many cases it is the wound itself that raises suspicion of malignancy; for example, when a patient who has no previous diagnosis of cancer presents with a wound that fails to heal a nurse may suspect malignancy so requests a biopsy that then confirms the diagnosis.

Suspecting a malignant wound

In these cases it is common for the patient to attend a nurse for wound dressings for many months and even years without any significant healing rate. This is because the underlying cause (i.e. cancer) has not been identified and addressed and so the wound is unable to heal.

Unless the nurse is aware of the common signs associated with these wound types the patient's condition can continue to be left untreated, to the patients detriment. A wound of significant longevity that fails to heal must be therefore be referred to and reassessed by a specialist for further investigations into why the wound is failing to heal. This could be to a tissue viability nurse or a doctor in the first instance, and then to a dermatologist for wound biopsy or other investigations in the second. It is common practice to refer to a tissue viability nurse or a doctor (GP) any patient with a wound that fails to heal or progresses towards healing within 6 weeks. In that time the nurse would be expected to adhere to the best practices in wound management as described in this book. If a nurse is highly suspicious of malignancy in a wound before this time, it is wise to make this referral sooner than the aforementioned 6-week timeframe.

Common signs of a malignant wound

The most suspicious signs are the lack of identifiable causes and the wound's failure to heal. The malignant wound is often very perfectly round in shape; the tissue on the wound bed often alters shape and size very quickly (from one day to the next) and is often mistaken for hypergranulating tissue (discussed in other chapters) (Figure 48.3), not least due to its cauliflower appearance and friable tissue that bleeds easily. The wound is often painless and/or itchy. Occasionally a wound may heal then recur again in a cyclic manner. These symptoms in themselves do not confirm a malignant wound but should raise the suspicions of the assessing nurse.

As the disease within the wound progresses, the symptoms become more obvious in terms of increased exudate levels, a more profound, larger wound with tissue that sits more proud than the surrounding skin and the wound will often bleed very easily. There may be a malodour and the patient may complain of increasing pain or loss of function, particularly on a limb. Lymphoedema may occur as can be seen in Figure 48.1. Prompt referral and diagnosis is essential in these cases.

Management of the malignant wound

First and foremost, a medical diagnosis will be required to determine whether or not the wound is malignant. In many cases the patient can be treated to eliminate the cancer; however, in many cases there is no treatment available and it will be a nurse's responsibility to monitor and manage the following symptoms sufficiently to enable the patient to achieve an optimum quality of life.

Exudate management – all wounds will produce exudate, and malignant wounds are no exception. Indeed this type of wound often produces excessive amounts of exudate due to the underlying destruction of lymph glands and other underlying tissues, making the wound the easiest route for the escape of other bodily fluids. As the exudate levels increase, so bacteria will be provided with an optimum environment to multiply in, and so the exudate levels increase, and the cycle continues. Often patients become isolated because they fear the embarrassment of exudate leakage when they are in the company of others

Malodour – as a result of increased bacterial growth, a malodour will occur (bacteria are living creatures who pass flatus as with any other living creature). The higher the levels of bacteria the greater the malodour will be, thereby isolating the patient further.

Pain – Many malignant wounds are very painful for the patient and effective assessment and monitoring of pain levels and efficacy of analgesics is crucial to promote an acceptable pain level for the patient. Pain can be exacerbated by inappropriate and ineffectual exudate management, as bacteria and fungus will rapidly increase in a wet environment. The waste products from the bacteria alter the pH value within the exudate making the tissues (and nerve endings) more sensitive as a result of this change in environment.

Given the above symptoms it is clear that effective exudate management will reduce and minimize the other two symptoms in turn. Therefore, timely dressing changes, and appropriate dressing selection (see Dressing selection guide) is crucial in maintaining a reasonable quality of life for the patient.

49 Palliative wound care

Palliative care is a term used when the patient's disease is no longer responsive to treatments and the condition is rendering the patient more and more debilitated as they approach the end of their life. Patients in this situation often either have existing wounds as a result of their terminal condition (e.g. surgical wounds or fungating ulcers) or they develop unavoidable wounds (e.g. pressure ulcers) as a result of their declining general health. By nature of the underlying causative disease, they are likely to have significant pain levels to deal with and the presence of a wound can add to those pain levels if not adequately managed. In many cases of palliative care it is improbable that a wound will heal, and chances are that it will get larger, and so the aim of treating wounds in these patients changes from promoting healing to managing and controlling the symptoms associated with wounds, and as far as possible preventing deterioration. That is not to say our aims should not include creating the right wound conditions that would promote healing if it were possible, but simply states that our priorities and expectations must change for the sake of the patients comfort and quality of life. Many wounds will heal in the end of life stages if we apply appropriate wound management. However, inappropriate wound management could hasten the death of the patient and is unacceptable.

Priorities in wound care

As always, a nursing priority is to assess the patient holistically taking into consideration the physical, psychological, emotional, environmental and social aspects affecting the patient. In particular, consideration must be given to the patient's nutritional status, mobility, site of the wound and the patients (substantial) potential for infection, as well as assessing the pain levels experienced by the patient in order to prescribe treatments that will meet their needs whilst minimising or reducing the patients pain.

Pressure ulcer prevention – there is much debate regarding the ethical issues relating to the development or deterioration of pressure ulcers in the terminally ill patient, and so care must be carefully planned in conjunction with the patient so that repositioning intervals can be agreed that is within their individual tolerance levels and that the most suitable pressure relieving devices can be used to adequately achieve the agreed repositioning regime. Very small frequent position changes can be acceptable to patients rather than one complete change from one side to the other every 2 hours or so. This can be achieved by moving the patient gradually at smaller angles and at shorter intervals from one side to the other until the patient has reached the 30° tilt on one side then the other. If this is done in conjunction with appropriate equipment (e.g. a low-air-loss mattress and a profiling bed), this may be acceptable to a patient and will minimize the risk of pressure ulcer development. However, in many cases pressure damage will occur despite our best efforts, due to the failing nature of the patient's general health, and particularly if the patient is unable to tolerate such a repositioning regime.

Pain – is the most distressing symptom for the patient and their loved ones who observe the patients distress. Pain can be multifactorial and can be caused by the terminal illness itself, the effects of pressure on the skin, exposed nerve endings on an open wound,

inappropriate use of dressings, poor wound care techniques and increasing levels of bacteria on a wound.

Wound infection – all wounds will have bacteria or fungi growing on the wound bed. As bacterial levels increase this alters the pH levels on the wound, which in turn irritates/causes pain to the exposed nerve endings. In the event of a wound infection extreme levels of pain can be experienced due to the spreading infection into localised tissues.

Malodour – many malignant and most, if not all infected wounds will omit an unpleasant odour. This is caused by the flatus of the microbes living on the wound. The odour may cause the patient to become isolated as they feel embarrassed so refuse to accept visitors, and this in turn reduces their quality of life. Malodours can be minimized and/or controlled with the provision of good wound care and so the patient should not experience such isolation.

Exudate management – all wounds will exude fluid (exudate) although in a healthy wound this is a minimal amount. In malignant wounds the exudate levels rise due to a number of reasons; the site of the wound (e.g. escape of lymph fluid); oedema due to poor cardiovascular circulation; and increased levels of bacteria/fungi that develop on the wound. If a wound becomes infected the exudate levels will be excessive, thereby reducing the quality of life for the patient. The amount of exudate can be extremely distressing and embarrassing for the patient and so exudate control can be extremely challenging for the nurse.

Topical treatments

The priorities in wound care therefore lie in the management of the following:

Pain – using non-adherent dressings will minimize pain on dressing removal. If a dressing has adhered to a wound this ought to be soaked thoroughly with saline so that it can be removed without causing pain or trauma. Taking note and reacting to signs of critical colonisation or infection in a timely manner using antimicrobial dressings will reduce pain levels for patients. In some cases of palliative care only, topical analgesics are applied (e.g. morphine gels); however, this must only be done under medical or palliative care specialist advice.

Wound infection – topical sustained release antimicrobials (e.g. silver impregnated dressings) in conjunction with antibiotics (if deemed appropriate) will assist in eliminating the wound infection. The ideal would be to prevent infection occurring in the first instance by applying prophylactic antimicrobial dressings or by applying them in a timely manner on recognition of signs of critical colonisation (increased pain/tenderness and increased exudate levels).

Malodour – as with the recommendations for wound infection, topical antimicrobials will kill bacteria that are causing the odour. Charcoal dressings can be used as they will absorb the odour thereby making it more acceptable to the patient and loved ones. However, the nurse must be mindful that this will not eliminate the cause of the odour and so antimicrobials will be necessary as well as charcoal dressings.

Exudate – highly absorbent dressings such as foam, or wound drainage bags can be used along with timely dressing changes to reduce the environment for bacterial growth and further tissue destruction caused by maceration.

Wound Care at a Glance, First Edition. Ian Peate and Wyn Glencross. © 2015 John Wiley & Sons, Ltd. Published 2015 by John Wiley & Sons, Ltd.
Companion website: www.ataglanceseries.com/nursing/woundcare

Glossary

Abrasion A wearing away of the skin through some mechanical process, such as friction or trauma

Abscess A circumscribed collection of pus that forms in tissue as a result of acute or chronic localised infection and is associated with tissue destruction and, in many cases, swelling

Acute wound Any wound that's new or progressing as expected

Alginate A non-woven, highly absorptive dressing that's manufactured from seaweed (kelp)

Angiogenesis The formation and regeneration of blood vessels

Antimicrobial An agent that kills microbes or inhibits their growth

Autolysis The breakdown of tissues or cells by the body's own mechanisms, such as enzymes or white blood cells

Bacteria One-celled microorganisms that break down dead tissue; they have no true nucleus and reproduce by cell division

Blanchable erythema A reddened area of the skin that temporarily turns white or pale when pressure is applied with a fingertip

Burn An acute wound caused by exposure to thermal extremes, electricity, radiation or caustic chemicals

Cellulitis An infection of the deeper layers of the skin and the underlying tissue

Chemical debridement Application, topically, of biological enzymes to break down devitalised tissue

Chronic wound A wound where healing is slow or stopped it does not heal in a timely fashion

Collagen A supportive protein of skin, bone, tendon, connective tissue and cartilage

Colonized A wound contaminated with bacteria

Debridement Removal of necrotic tissue providing the underlying healthy tissue to regenerate

Debris The remains of damaged cells or tissues

Dehiscence Complication of wound healing where the wound may fully or partially open up

Dermis The inner thick layer of the skin

Enzyme A protein that acts as a catalyst causing chemical changes to occur

Epidermis The skins outer most layer

Epithelization Regeneration of skin across the surface of a wound

Erythema Redness of the skin cause by the engorgement of the capillaries

Eschar Dead wound tissue appears as a dry leathery crust

Evisceration The protrusion of an visceral organ from a wound

Excoriation Skin abrasions

Exudate Any fluid that filters from the circulatory system into lesions or areas of inflammation

Fascia A layer of fibrous tissue

Fibrin An insoluble protein formed from fibrinogen during the clotting of blood, forming a fibrous mesh, impeding the flow of blood

Fibroblasts A type of cell that synthesizes the extracellular matrix and collagen, the structural framework for tissues, plays a central role in healing wounds. Fibroblasts are the most common cells of connective tissue

Full thickness wound A penetrating wound completely through the skin protruding through the underlying tissues, bone may be exposed

Granulation Occurs where new connective tissue and tiny blood vessels form on the surfaces of a wound during the healing process. Typically granulation tissue grows from the base of a wound and is able to fill almost any size of wound

Hydrocolloid A wafer type of dressing containing gel-forming agents in an adhesive compound laminated onto a flexible, water-resistant outer layer. Some types include an alginate to increase absorption capabilities

Hydrogel A water based none adherent type of dressing with some ability to absorb

Hydrophilic Has the ability to attract water – readily absorbs moisture

Hypoxia Reduction in the amount of oxygen reaching the tissues

Induration A process where the skin becomes firm, often surrounds a wound as a healing ridge

Inflammation This is a localize protective response causes heat, redness, swelling, pain and loss of function. During this phase the body attempts to close off broken blood vessels and clean up the wound

Ischaemia A deficiency of blood supply to an area

Keloid A type of scar that is often red and prominent. It is caused by excessive collagen formation in the corium during connective tissue repair

Keratin An insoluble protein forming the principal component of epidermis, hair, nails and tooth enamel

Leucocytes The colourless blood corpuscles whose chief function is to protect the body against micro-organisms

Lymphocyte A mononuclear, non-granular leucocyte, chiefly a product of lymphoid tissue, which participates in the immune response

Lymphoedema A swelling that develops as a result of an impaired lymphatic system

Maceration A softening and whitish look to the intact skin around wounds caused by excessive moisture. Often occurs when exudate is not well managed by dressings

Macrophage Any of the large, mononuclear, phagocytotic cells derived from monocytes that are found in the walls of blood vessels and in loose connective tissue. They become stimulated by inflammation on initial angiogenesis

Matrix The intracellular substance of a tissue that forms the framework of tissues

Maturation A phase in wound healing where scar tissue is remodelled

Mechanical debridement The removal of dead or devitalized tissue by use of wet to dry dressings, whirlpool, lavage or scrubbing (for example with gauze)

Myofibroblast A differentiated fibroblast containing the ultrastructural features of a fibroblast and a smooth muscle cell containing many actin-rich microfilaments

Necrosis Death of tissue or cell

Neutrophil White blood cell responsible for phagocytosis

Non-blanching erythema Redness of the skin persisting when gentle pressure is applied and then released

Occlusive dressing A dressing that closes the wound from the external environment

Pathogen An organism that can cause disease such as a virus, bacteria or other micro-organism

Phagocytosis The process where cells surround and digest cell debris, micro-organisms necrotic tissue and foreign bodies

Proliferation The growth or reproduction of tissue as part of the healing process

Pus A thick yellowish fluid composed of dead bacteria and leucocytes

Purulent Containing or pus forming

Scab Dry crust forming over an open wound, consists of skin and debris

Septicaemia Blood poisoning: a systemic disease where pathogenic micro-organisms are present and multiply in the blood

Slough Dead tissue often yellow in colour and can be stringy in appearance

Suppuration Formation of discharge or pus

Suture A stitch or series of stitches made to secure the opposition of the edges of a surgical or a traumatic wound

Tensile strength The strength of a closed or healed wound in terms of the greatest stress the tissues can bear without tearing

Wound Any break in the skin

References and further reading

Baranoski, S. (2012) *Wound Care Essentials: Practice and Principles.* 3rd Ed. Philadelphia: Lippincott.

Bale, S. (2006) *Wound Care Nursing: A Patient Centred Approach.* 2nd Ed. Edinburgh: Elsevier.

Bryant, R.A. and Nix, D.P. (2012) *Acute and Chronic Wounds: Current Management Concepts.* 4th Ed. St Louis: Mosby.

Davey, P. (2014). *Medicine at a Glance.* 4th Ed. Oxford: John Wiley & Sons, Ltd.

Dealey, C. (2012) *The Care of Wounds: A Guide for Nurses.* 4th Ed. Philadelphia: Lippincott.

Dorresteijn, J. et al. (2010) Patient education for preventing diabetic foot ulceration. *Cochrane Database of Systematic Reviews*, Issue 5, Art No: CD001488. doi:10.1002/14651858.CD001488.pub3

Dougherty, L. and Lister S. (2011) *The Royal Marsden Hospital Manual of Clinical Nursing Procedures.* 8th Ed. Oxford: Wiley-Blackwell.

Flanagan, M. (2000) The physiology of wound healing. *Journal of Wound Care* 9(6): 299–300.

Flanagan, M. (2013) *Wound Healing and Skin Integrity.* Oxford: Wiley.

Foster, J.G. (2012) *Management of Complex Wounds.* Philadelphia: Saunders.

Grey, J.E., Harding, K.G. and Enoch, S. (2006) ABC of wound healing: Pressure ulcers. *BMJ* 332:472–475.

Keast, D.H. et al. (2004) MEASURE: A proposed assessment framework for developing best practice recommendations for wound assessment. *Wound Repair and Regeneration* 12: S1–S17.

Lawenda, B.D., Mondry, T.E. and Johnstone, P.A.S. (2009). Lymphedema: A primer on the identification and management of a chronic condition in oncologic treatment. *CA: A Cancer Journal for Clinicians* 59: 8–24.

The Malnutrition Advisory Group (2004). *Malnutrition Universal Screening Tool (MUST).* Redditch: BAPEN.

Moffatt, C., Marin, R. and Smithdale, R. (2007) *Leg Ulcer Management.* Oxford: Blackwell.

Moore, K. (2005) Using wound area measurement to predict and monitor response to treatment of chronic wounds. *Journal of Wound Care* 14(5): 229–232.

Myers, B.A. (2012) *Wound Management: Principles and Practice.* 3rd Ed. New Jersey: Pearson.

Mudge, E. and Orsted, H. (2010) Wound infection and pain management made easy. *Wounds International* 1(3). http://www.woundsinternational.com/pdf/content_8902.pdf

Nair, M. and Peate, I. (2013). *Fundamentals of Applied Pathophysiology.* 2nd Ed. Oxford: John Wiley & Sons, Ltd.

Onesti, M.G. et al. (2013). Ten years of experience in chronic ulcers and malignant transformation. *International Wound Journal.* doi:10.1111/iwj.12134

Ousey, K. (2007) *Lower Extremity Wounds: A Problem Based Learning Approach.* Oxford: Wiley.

Reynolds, V. (2013) Assessing and diagnosing wound infection (Part 1). *Nurse Prescribing* 11(3): 114–121.

Thomas, S. (2010) *Surgical Dressings and Wound Management.* Cardiff: Medetec.

Thompson, M. & Van den Bruel, A. (2011). *Diagnostic Tests Toolkit.* Oxford: John Wiley & Sons, Ltd.

Timmons, J. (2006). Skin function and wound healing physiology. *Wound Essentials*: 1: 8-17. http://www.wounds-uk.com/pdf/content_9363.pdf

Vowden, P., Vowden, K. and Carville, K. (2011) Antimicrobial dressing made easy. *Wounds International* 2(1). http://www.woundsinternational.com/made-easys/antimicrobial-dressings-made-easy

Ward, J.P.T. and Linden R.W.A. (2013). *Physiology at a Glance.* 3rd Ed. Oxford: John Wiley & Sons, Ltd.

Index